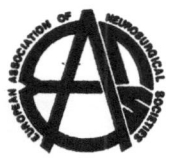

Sponsored by the
European Association of Neurosurgical Societies

Advances and Technical Standards in Neurosurgery

Edited by

H. Krayenbühl, Zürich (Managing Editor)
J. Brihaye, Bruxelles
F. Loew, Homburg/Saar
V. Logue, London
S. Mingrino, Padova
B. Pertuiset, Paris
L. Symon, London
H. Troupp, Helsinki
M. G. Yaşargil, Zürich

Volume **9**

Springer -Verlag
Wien New York 1982

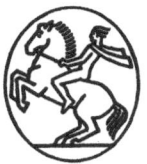

With 88 Figures

© 1982 by Springer-Verlag/Wien

Softcover reprint of the hardcover 1st edition 1982

Library of Congress Catalog Card Number 74-10499

ISSN 0095-4829

ISBN-13:978-3-7091-7036-6   e-ISBN-13:978-3-7091-7034-2

DOI: 10.1007/978-3-7091-7034-2

Preface

As an addition to the European postgraduate training system for young neurosurgeons we began to publish in 1974 this series devoted to Advances and Technical Standards in Neurosurgery which was later sponsored by the European Association of Neurosurgical Societies.

The fact that the English language is well on the way to becoming the international medium at European scientific conferences is a great asset in terms of mutual understanding. Therefore we have decided to publish all contributions in English, regardless of the native language of the authors.

All contributions are submitted to the entire editorial board before publication of any volume.

Our series is not intended to compete with the publications of original scientific papers in other neurosurgical journals. Our intention is, rather, to present fields of neurosurgery and related areas in which important recent advances have been made. The contributions are written by specialists in the given fields and constitute the first part of each volume.

In the second part of each volume, we publish detailed descriptions of standard operative procedures, furnished by experienced clinicians; in these articles the authors describe the techniques they employ and explain the advantages, difficulties and risks involved in the various procedures. This part is intended primarily to assist young neurosurgeons in their postgraduate training. However, we are convinced that it will also be useful to experienced, fully trained neurosurgeons.

The descriptions of standard operative procedures are a novel feature of our series which will be mainly, but not exclusively, a forum for European neurosurgeons. We intend as well to make available the findings of European neurosurgeons which are published in less familiar languages to neurosurgeons beyond the boundaries of the authors' countries and of Europe, and we aim to promote contacts among European neurosurgeons.

We hope that neurosurgeons not only in Europe, but throughout the world, will profit by this series of "Advances and Technical Standards in Neurosurgery".

The Editors

Contents

B. Technical Standards

X   Contents

List of Contributors

Faulhauer, Prof. Dr. K., Neurochirurgische Abteilung, Krankenhaus der Barmherzigen Brüder, D-5500 Trier, Federal Republic of Germany.

Loew, Prof. Dr. F., Neurochirurgische Universitätsklinik, D-6650 Homburg/Saar, Federal Republic of Germany.

Romodanov, Prof. Dr. A. P., Kiev Research Institute of Neurosurgery, Manuilsky St. 32, 252655 Kiev, USSR.

Shcheglov, Dr. V. I., Kiev Research Institute of Neurosurgery, Manuilsky St. 32, 252655 Kiev, USSR.

Spiess, PD Dr. H., Neuroradiologisches Institut, Talstrasse 65, CH-8001 Zürich, Switzerland.

Symon, Prof. Dr. L., Institute of Neurology, Gough-Cooper Department of Neurological Surgery, The National Hospital, Queen Square, London WC 1 E 3 BG, Great Britain.

Williams, Prof. Dr. B., The Midland Centre for Neurosurgery and Neurology, Holly Lane, Smethwick, Warley B 6 Z 8 BJ, Great Britain.

A. Advances

The Overdrained Hydrocephalus.
Clinical Manifestations and Management

K. Faulhauer

Neurochirurgische Abteilung, Krankenhaus der Barmherzigen Brüder, Trier
(Federal Republic of Germany)

With 11 Figures

Contents

I. Introduction

The history of the treatment of hydrocephalus is one of the most fascinating chapters in Neurosurgery. With the publication of the first successful clinical use of a one way valve by Nulsen and Spitz in 1952 a new era of hydrocephalus treatment started. The numerous approaches, techniques and operative trials have been meticuously compiled by Scarff (1963).

Since 1952 innumerable valve regulated CSF shunts have been produced. Aside from the obvious commercial aspects, the large variety of different catheters, valves and connectors seems to prove that the ideal shunt has not yet been developed.

Shunt operations still have the highest complication rate in Neurosurgery, infection or obstruction being in most cases the cause for shunt revision. The revision rate in recent papers varies between 1.74 and 4.34 operations per patient (Raimondi 1977, Keucher 1979).

Beside these two well-known complications there is a third category of undesirable side-effects, which are caused by CSF overdrainage. In many reports on long term results and complications in shunt surgery, these sequelae are either not mentioned at all (Steinbok 1976, Hemmer 1977, Keucher 1979) or inadequately considered (Raimondi 1977, Guidetti 1976). Guidetti for example conceded that his reported 5% subdural haematomas and 0.5% "excessive CSF drainage" did not reflect the real data. He felt that cases of overdrained hydrocephalus were definitely more numerous than his series implied. Raimondi, however, found only 5 subdural haematomas among 457 patients.

There has been a remarkable delay between the introduction of the modern valve regulated CSF shunts and the discovery of those different complications due to excessive CSF drainage.

Although some detailed aspects of the hyperdrainage problem have been mentioned quite frequently in the literature, only the most recent publications show a world wide general acceptance of this matter and offer some practical advice in handling these special complications. It is the objective of the author, to compile all the various clinical symptoms and radiological signs which derive from CSF hyperdrainage the to extracranial CSF shunts and to present practical suggestions for their management.

II. Theoretical Considerations

All extracranial shunting systems work on the basis of a differential pressure valve. It is not the intraventricular pressure itself but the pressure gradient between the ventricles and the body space to which CSF is diverted that determines CSF flow.

There have been quite a number of publications about the hydrodynamic properties and flow characteristics of different commercially available shunts (Rayport 1969, Hakim 1972, Fox 1973, Harbert 1974, McCullough 1974), but the applicability of such studies *in vivo* been has widely questioned.

It has also been shown in patients shunted for hydrocephalus, that in the erect position extraordinary low intracranial pressures, as low as -400 mm H_2O may occur (McCullough 1974, Portnoy 1973). These findings were confirmed by Shokei Yamada (1975) in animal experiments; the intraventricular pressure dropped to -120 mm water in shunted dogs brought into the upright position, whereas it remained in the positive range in the recumbent position. Ventriculopleural shunts in dogs with Kaolin induced hydrocephalus caused slit ventricles, promoted bulk flow from parenchyma to the ventricle and a diminution of diffusion from the ventricle into the brain (Ito, M. 1979).

Hiroshi Yamada (1975) investigated the effect of respiratory movements on the intracranial, atrial and peritoneal pressure. He was able to show that in the crying or straining child the pressure in the right atrium dropped to -100 to -200 mm H_2O, while intra-ventricular and peritoneal pressure remained above

0 mm H_2O. The intracranial pressure in shunted babies with cardiac diversion was significantly lower than in those with peritoneal shunts.

This adds to the well-known siphon effect a second cause for pressure gradients leading to undesired CSF drainage.

Practically, pressure gradients causing CSF flow through the shunting system, may arise from the following situations.

1. Increase of CSF pressure, which would be the clinical situation for which the system was designed;

2. Negative pressure waves in the right atrium caused by profound ventilation and

3. Siphon effects of the distal catheter in the upright position.

No present-day extracranial CSF shunts with their low or high resistance valves are able to distinguish between positive pressure in the CSF space and negative pressure in the distal space. There is no need to stress the point that negative pressure affecting the valve distally as caused by the above mentioned mechanisms is probably active in every case. The minimal threshold usually offered by the valvular resistance can easily be overcome by these negative forces resulting finally in a subnormal intracranial pressure.

III. Clinical Manifestations

The symptomatology of overdrained hydrocephalus is quite varied and depends on many factors such as the patients age, the degree of ventricular dilatation, the grade of siphon effect and the extent of substantial brain damage. Are the fontanelles open or are the sutures closed? Is the patient mainly in the horizontal position as in the baby or the unconscious, or does he live normally, sitting, walking and standing i.e. in the upright position? The clinical picture extends between an acute, severe and sometimes fatal disease and a harmless, symptomfree condition, discovered incidently in an X-ray study.

1. Acute Decompression

Over-rapid decompression of a large hydrocephalus may cause an acute clinical syndrome with vegetative signs such as tachycardia, pallor, peripheral vasoconstriction, headaches, irritability, stiffness of the neck and changes of sensorium and consciousness. These symptoms are caused by upward displacement of the brain stem. In many instances such conditions are due to uncontrolled loss of CSF during operation. They may however also happen in appropriately shunted patients. In his analysis of over 60 autopsies of shunt treated children, Emery (1965) describes the upward movement of the brain stem associated with lifting of the hypothalamus and stretching of the pituitary stalk. Confronted by such a severe and alarming postoperative clinical condition, it is not easy to differentiate between an acute haematoma, shunt malfunction or negative pressure problems. In small children with open fontanelles diagnosis is easy. When the cranial sutures are closed CT-scan and puncture of the valvechamber will help to elucidate the situation.

2. Microcrania, Craniostenosis

In smaller children with open sutures a marked reduction of CSF volume and ventricular size after shunt operation is normal and desirable. This volume decrease clearly shows in the head circumference curve. Besides the slow approximation to the normal we often see a rapid decline into the microcephalic range. In babies the rapid and excessive drainage of large ventricles causes the well-known clinical picture of deeply sunken fontanelle, overriding of the cranial bones and finally because of the lateral recumbent positioning of the babies mostly dolichocephalic and rarely brachycephalic deformation of the skull. In

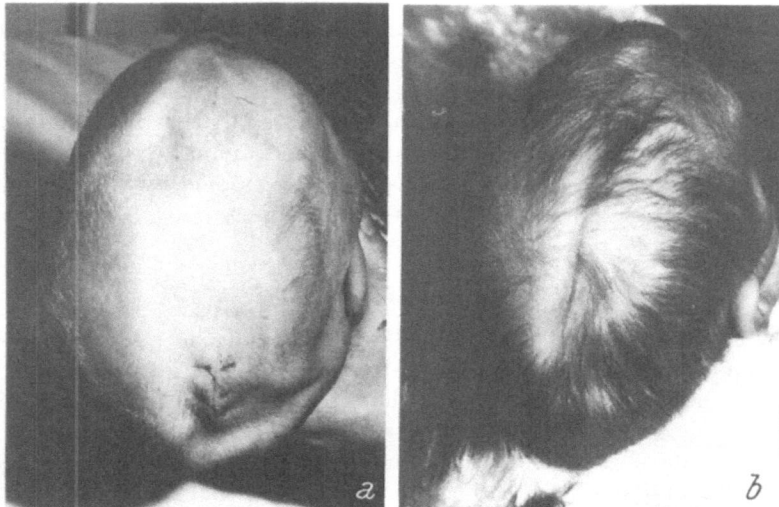

Fig. 1. (a) Acute decompression. Deeply sunken fontanelle, overriding of the parietal bones. (b) The same child a few weeks later

this sometimes grotesque deformation the skull consolidates because of premature synostosis. The skull deformation is also irreversible because surgical opening of the sutures does not help to normalize the cranial appearance when hyperdrainage of CSF persists. These misshapen heads are not a cosmetic problem, they also indicate the simultaneous evacuation of the spatial buffer represented mainly by the cerebro-spinal fluid.

In our series (400 patients) 33 of the shunted babies developed marked microcrania (distinctly below the 5th percentile). Eighteen of these had scaphocephaly with synostosis of the sagittal suture. The other cases had oxy- or brachycephaly (Faulhauer 1978).

Craniosynostosis secondary to ventriculo-atrial shunt was the first complication which was clearly recognized and related to CSF overdrainage (Anderson 1966, Kloss 1968 and Roberts 1970).

Roberts and Rickham (1970) saw 8 cases of craniostenosis in 800 operated children. Because these cases showed considerable destruction of brain tissue

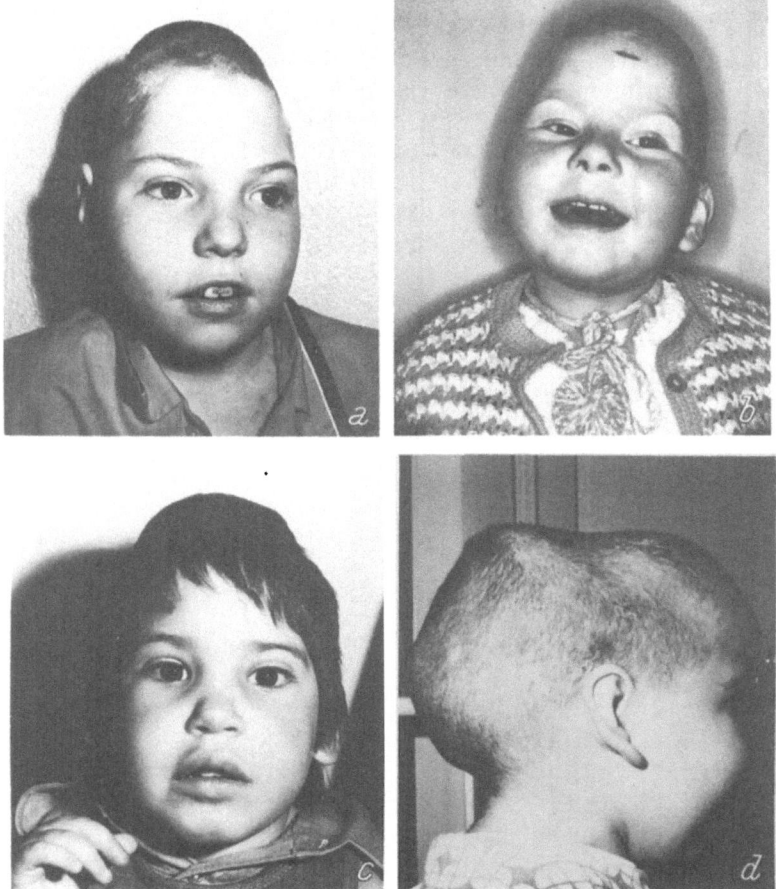

Fig. 2 a–d. Scaphocephalic head deformation in three different children. (d) (same child as c) shows typical head deformation due to stenosis of the coronal suture

secondary to severe hydrocephalus, they concluded that this complication indicated a poor prognosis.

Since almost all cases of craniostenosis were reported to have low pressure valves, Anderson (1966) and Kloss (1968) decided to use medium pressure valves.

In 1976 Hoffman described 8 cases who developed small heads following treatment with lumbo-peritoneal shunts. Despite demonstrated shunt patency they showed on a later occasion signs of cerebellar herniation. They were successfully treated by posterior fossa decompression. The authors stated that skull growth was largely determined by the volumetric expansion of the brain. Continuous subnormal intracranial pressure resulted in an arrest of skull growth and finally secondary synostosis. When brain volume exceeded the available space the result was a state of "cephalocranial disproportion", which in some cases might lead to foramen magnum impaction.

Craniostenosis is only one aspect of the many possible skull changes. Systematic descriptions of these changes were given by Griscom (1970), Kaufman (1973) and Villani (1976). Griscom aptly entitled the radiological sequels of hyperdrainage as contracting skull. The changes on plain skull X-ray

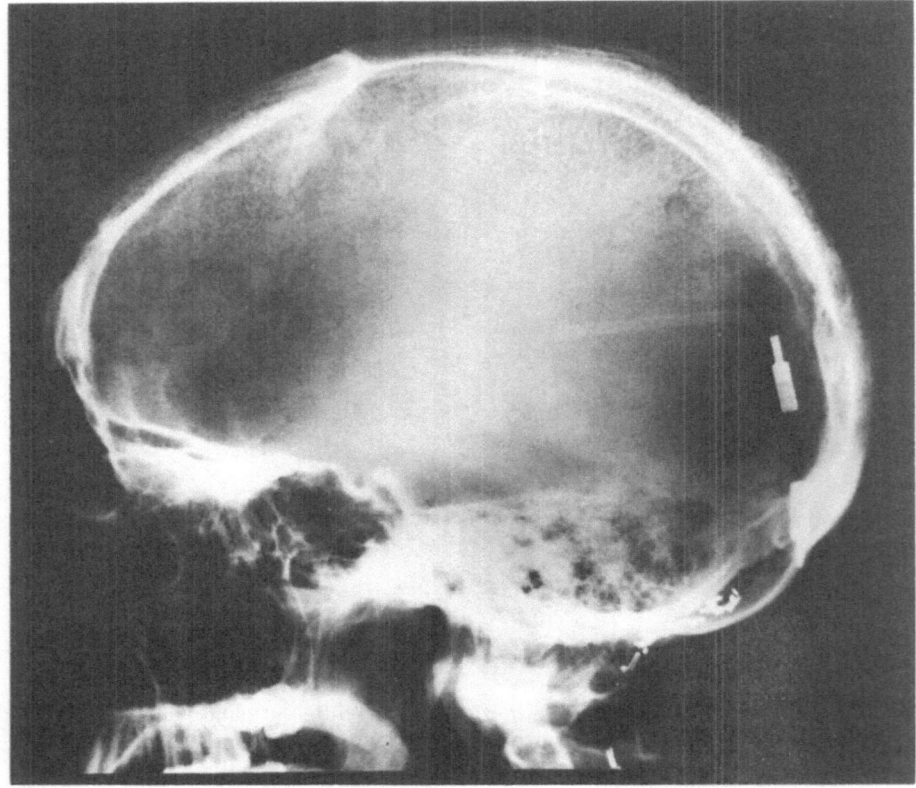

Fig. 3. Lateral view of the skull of a 13-year-old boy with long-standing extracranial drainage. Note extremely small sella, thickening of the cranial bone and hyper-pneumatized sinuses

can be summarized as follows: 1. microcrania and skull deformities, 2. premature synostoses, 3. thickening of the cranial bones and endocranial growth of the lamina interna, 4. hyperpneumatized sinuses and mastoids, 5. small sella and diminution of the foramina of the cranial nerves.

All these changes indicate a reduction of the intracranial capacity due to extracranial CSF drainage.

3. Collapsed or Slit Ventricles

Another problem arises from the contraction of the shunted ventricle, and this is quite common as we now know from computerized tomography. Close contact of the ventricular wall with the catheter favours occlusion of the catheter. Fortunately not all cases of over drained small ventricles are followed by ventricular catheter obstruction. Other factors like foreign body reaction and infection may be of some importance in the development of this complication.

In Torkildsen's ventriculo-cisternostomies ventricular catheter occlusions are almost unknown, conclusively proving that in the aetiology of this complication a foreign body reaction is of minor importance (Kirch 1977).

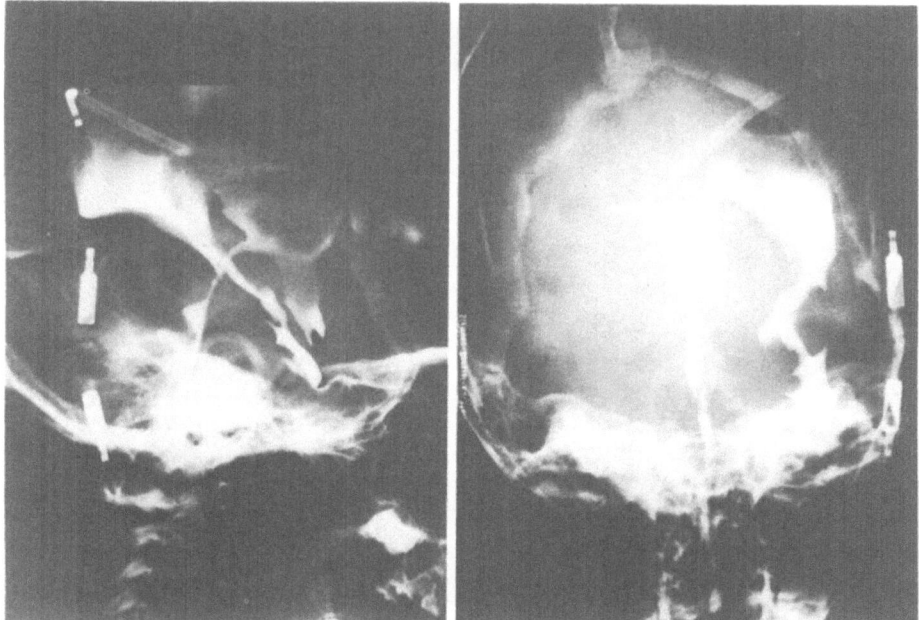

Fig. 4. "Slit ventricles" in positive ventriculography. Note the bizarre appearance of the contracted ventricles

In our 97 cases of ventricular catheter occlusion ventricular contraction was certainly one of the most prominent causes. In 12 cases recurrent catheter occlusion led to the clinical diagnosis of slit ventricle, mainly because of the difficulty of localizing the ventricle during the operation. In one case of repeated catheter occlusions an unintentional third ventriculostomy with placement of the catheter in the cisterna interpeducularis definitely helped the patient. In another case we were unable to find the ventricles and we had to perform a bitemporal decompression, as suggested by Epstein (1974).

In addition we have seen five children, who intermittently showed the picture of increased intracranial pressure. We think that in these cases complete occlusion of the ventricular catheter led to dilatation of the ventricles, and this again causes opening of some of the perforations of the catheter. Contrast medium studies in these cases seem to prove such a theory (Faulhauer 1978, Schmitz 1979).

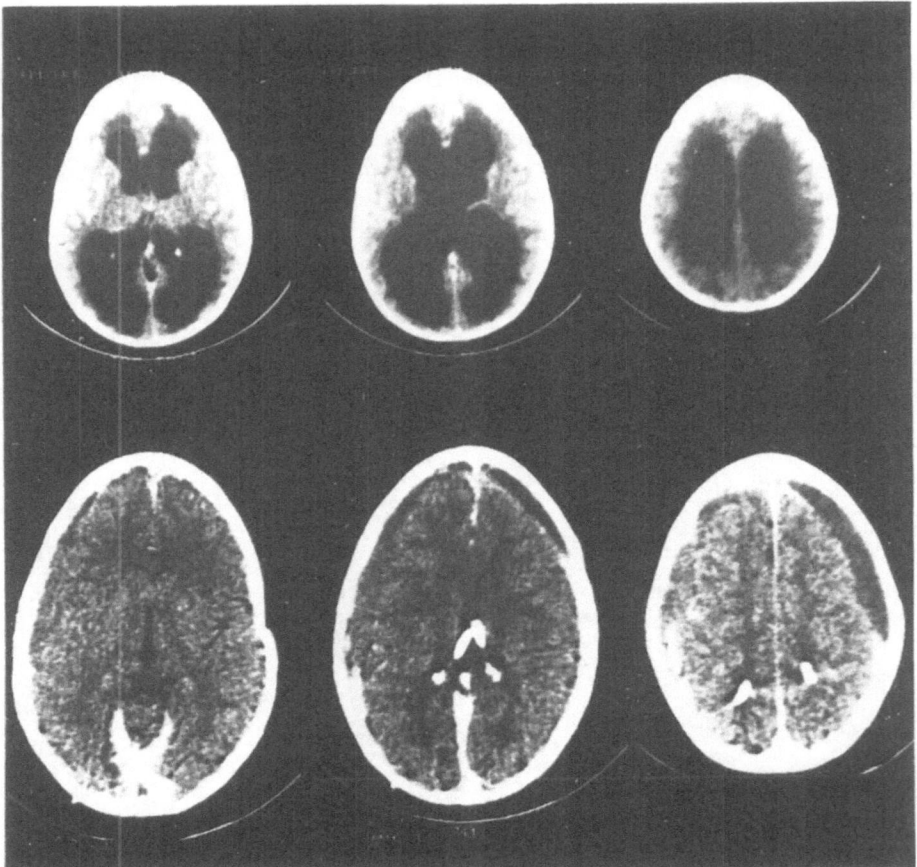

Fig. 5. "Slit ventricles" and bilateral subdural effusions (lower line) after peritoneal
drainage of large ventricles using a medium pressure valve

In 1974 Epstein described the slit ventricle syndrome in a paper about
"recurrent shunt obstruction secondary to small ventricles". His experience
with this desperate problem will lead to much experimental and clinical work on
shunt dependency. In a later publication in 1977 Epstein reported CCT follow-
up studies in shunted patients: he found that patients with normal or subnormal
ventricles tended to shunt dependency. In his article about management and
prevention of collapsed ventricles Salmon (1978) describes the clinical picture of
intermittent obstruction of the ventricular catheter: in the child with open
fontanelles the pressure episode is less dramatic than in the older patient with
rigid skull. In 1978 Moseley presented the results of 640 CCTs on 365 patients
with shunted hydrocephalus: patients deteriorating, with persistent headache or
suspected shunt malfunction showed increased tendency to persistent hydrocephalus, but recurrent ventricular dilatation was excluded in one third and 5%

showed collapsed ventricles. Meese (1976) had CCT controls on 125 shunted patients. Ventricular collapse was noted in 30%. In 1978 Venes found small ventricles in CCT controls of 7 (19%) out of 36 children presenting with shunt malfunction. She stated that slit ventricles in CCT may be more apparent than real, because in one case with slit ventricles, air injection in the shunt tube revealed normal sized ventricles. She overlooked that a "blown up" ventricle in air study is less real than the *in situ* picture of CCT.

4. Intolerance of CSF Pressure Elevation, Shunt Dependency

Patients with long-standing, excessive CSF drainage may become extremely sensitive to minimal intracranial pressure rises. In these patients an increase of CSF pressure within the normal range may cause clinical pressure symptoms up to respiratory arrest.

In our analysis of 400 shunted patients we have found 9 cases with such adaptive disturbances.

Four of these were connected to a pressure-controlled external CSF drainage (one patient because of valve infection and ventriculitis, three patients on account of the treatment of subdural haematoma). In five more patients the occlusion of the distal shunt catheter produced severe clinical pressure signs. The recording of ventricular pressure however, showed normal pressure values within the range of 50 to 150 mm H_2O (Faulhauer and Schmitz, 1978, 1979).

Epstein (1973) defined "shunt dependent" children as those with small ventricles, who are incapable of tolerating a minor degree of increased intracranial pressure. Therefore, this neurosurgical group did a great deal of work to make hydrocephalic patients shunt independent. It is doubtless to their credit that many neurosurgeons changed their minds about the need for permanently functioning CSF shunt. Consequently, some authors checked the shunt function of their patients and found in 20 to 30% arrested hydrocephalus (Holtzer 1973, Hayden 1974, Faulhauer 1975).

As mentioned above, there is much evidence that evacuation of the cranial CSF spaces is the main reason for the dangerous pressure sensitivity which in fact is mostly combined with microcrania, slit ventricles and other signs of hyperdrainage. Hoffman's 8 cases of cephalocranial disproportion in whom hindbrain herniation occurred despite normal shunt function probably also would have been extremely sensitive to minimal pressure rises.

As Epstein (1975) stated, shunt dependency may occur with either large or small ventricles. In fact in our pressure intolerant patients, there have been two with large ventricles and heads (Schmitz 1979), so that there must be additional mechanisms responsible for this serious problem.

5. Subdural Haematoma

Chronic subdural haematoma or subdural effusion is thought to be the most severe sequel of excessive CSF drainage, but this is true only for real space-occupying and not for space-filling haematomas and effusions. We found in 17 of our cases subdural haematomas, effusions, or callus. In addition, there was one case of epidural haematoma. Six subdural haematomas were discovered within the last two years by routine computerized tomography. In seven cases the diagnosis has been established more casually after demonstration of capsular calcification in the skull X-ray, typical findings in the brain scan. or accidentally during operative revision of the shunting system. This experience shows that subdural effusion in shunted patients in most instances does not cause specific

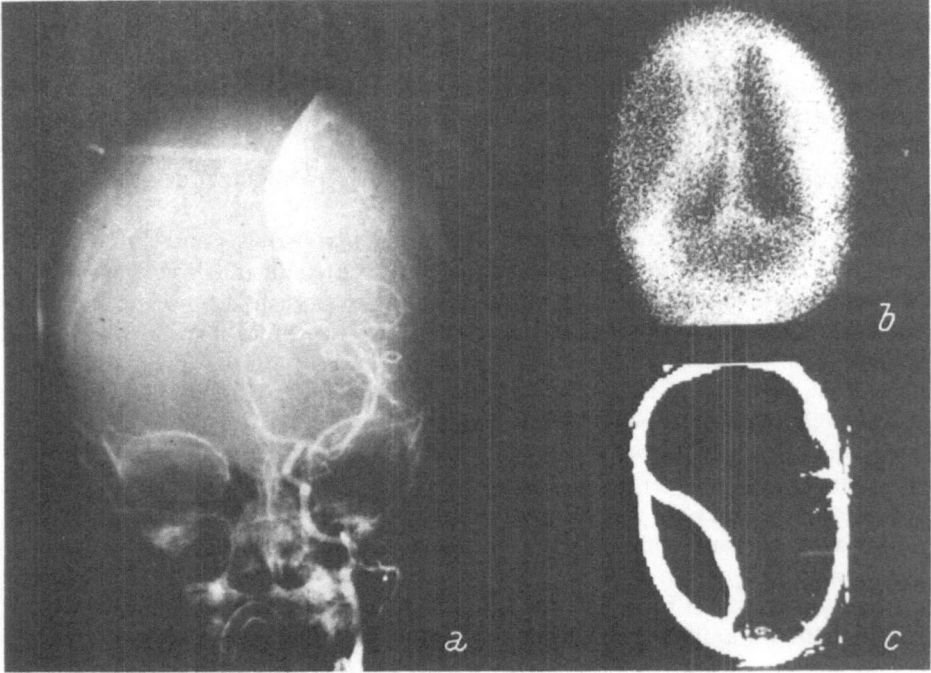

Fig. 6. Calcified chronic subdural haematoma: (a) angiography, (b) isotope scan, (c) CCT

clinical symptomatology, and that its discovery is frequently accidental. We therefore presume that in our patient material the incidence of subdural effusion in shunt treated patients may be even higher (Faulhauer 1978, Schmitz 1979).

In 1952 Anderson noted the relation between overdrainage and haematoma in three cases. After that more reports were published in literature. Becker and Nulsen (1968) had had 7 cases among 140 patients (5%). Illingworth (1970) found 8 haematoma patients in 175 cases (4,5%). Samuelson (1972) has published a remarkably high rate of secondary subdural haematomas (21%) following shunting procedures for normal pressure hydrocephalus. In the older publications (Forrest 1968, Shurtleff 1975) this complication is almost never mentioned. This is probably due to the fact that many secondary subdural effusions stay asymptomatic. Only nowadays, thanks to easy screening tests like brain scan

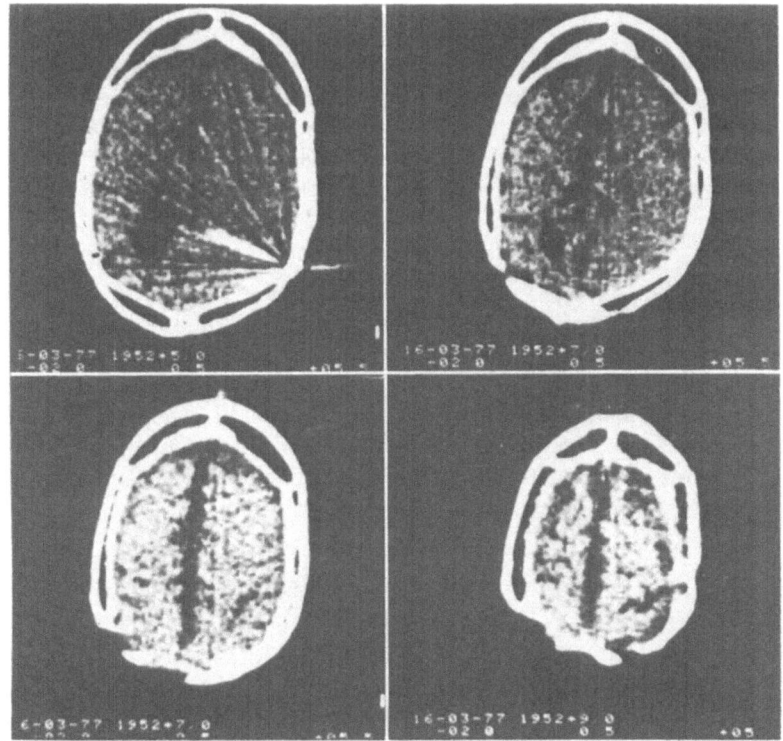

Fig. 7. Computerized tomography of a 15-year-old girl, who has developed a second
"inner skull" to adapt her cranial vault to the reduced intracranial volume

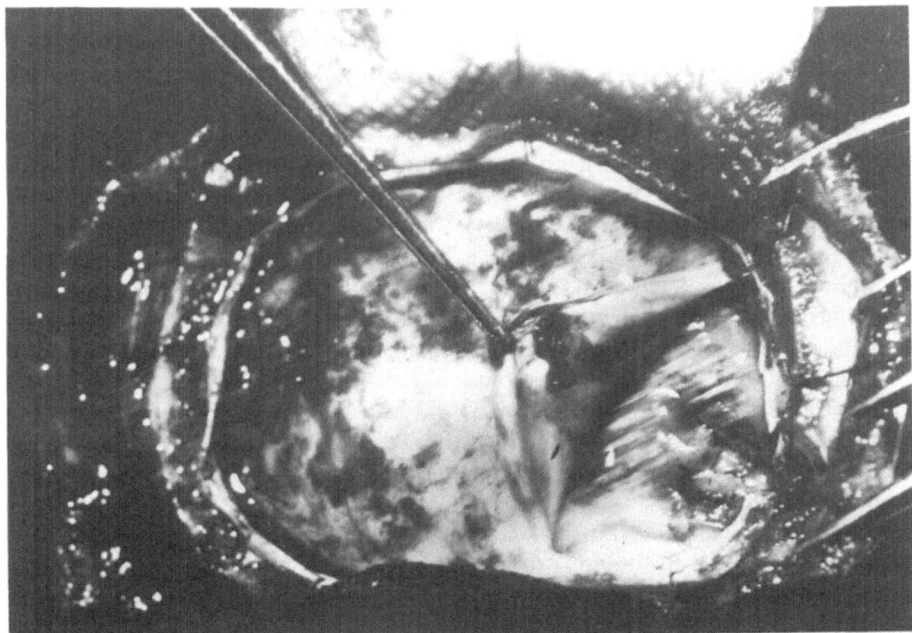

Fig. 8. Operative exposure of a post-shunt chronic subdural haematoma, which consisted
a thick capsule containing solid, callous-like material

and computerized tomography, can the real incidence be estimated. Meese (1976) reported 24% in 125 and Moseley (1978) 14% in 365 cases.

From clinical and especially therapeutic reasons it is important to distinguish space-filling from space-occupying subdural haematomas and effusions. Only real space-occupying haematomas and effusions need operative treatment.

6. Low Pressure Headaches

Headaches are only a minor problem because in most instances they disappear rapidly. Persistent headaches were complained of by 13 patients and in some cases nausea and vomiting were present. Diagnosis was proved by measuring the ventricular pressure in the flat and upright position (Faulhauer 1978). Jackson (1955) has pointed out, that headaches were observed in many children who had received peritoneal shunts but they were soon asymptomatic as they became adjusted to the low intracranial pressure. Guidetti (1976) has observed many cases of orthostatic headaches.

IV. Management of Overdrainage Symptoms

In the past many of us were concerned about keeping the shunts working. How they work and particularly the possible effects of overdrainage were secondary questions. But more and more as the management of hydrocephalus with extracranial diversions has become routine, the question of quality of drainage has come into general concern. Once the different complications due to excessive CSF flow were recognized, practical suggestions in handling these problems were published.

There is no big problem in handling the *acute postoperative decompression symptoms* by lowering the head as is also done in the immediate postoperative period in babies when deeply sunken fontanelles indicate undue negative intracranial pressure.

Microcrania, craniostenosis, cranio-cerebral disproportion, slit ventricles and intolerance of pressure rises are the main features of shunt dependency. None of these symptoms itself is sufficient motivation for real concern. However, the threatening danger of acute cerebral decompensation in cases of shunt malfunction and the simultaneous tendency of repeated ventricular catheter occlusion explain why some authors have given this syndrome a great deal of attention (Epstein, Hochwald). Reporting upon *craniostenosis* following shunt surgery some authors have felt that surgical correction of premature synostosis must be offered (Roberts 1970). He, however saw only initial improvement and gave a poor prognosis as to the ultimate outcome. Anderson (1966) warned about the complications in these operations and Hemmer (1966) did not feel the need to operate on the synostosis cases as long as the drainage worked well. Nowadays nobody would consider surgical correction of an X-ray finding like craniostenosis because after all the skull has adapted to the decreased intracranial volume and when the CSF drainage is functioning even after opening the sutures, the skull will not grow anymore.

When Epstein in 1974 published the subtemporal craniectomy for recurrent

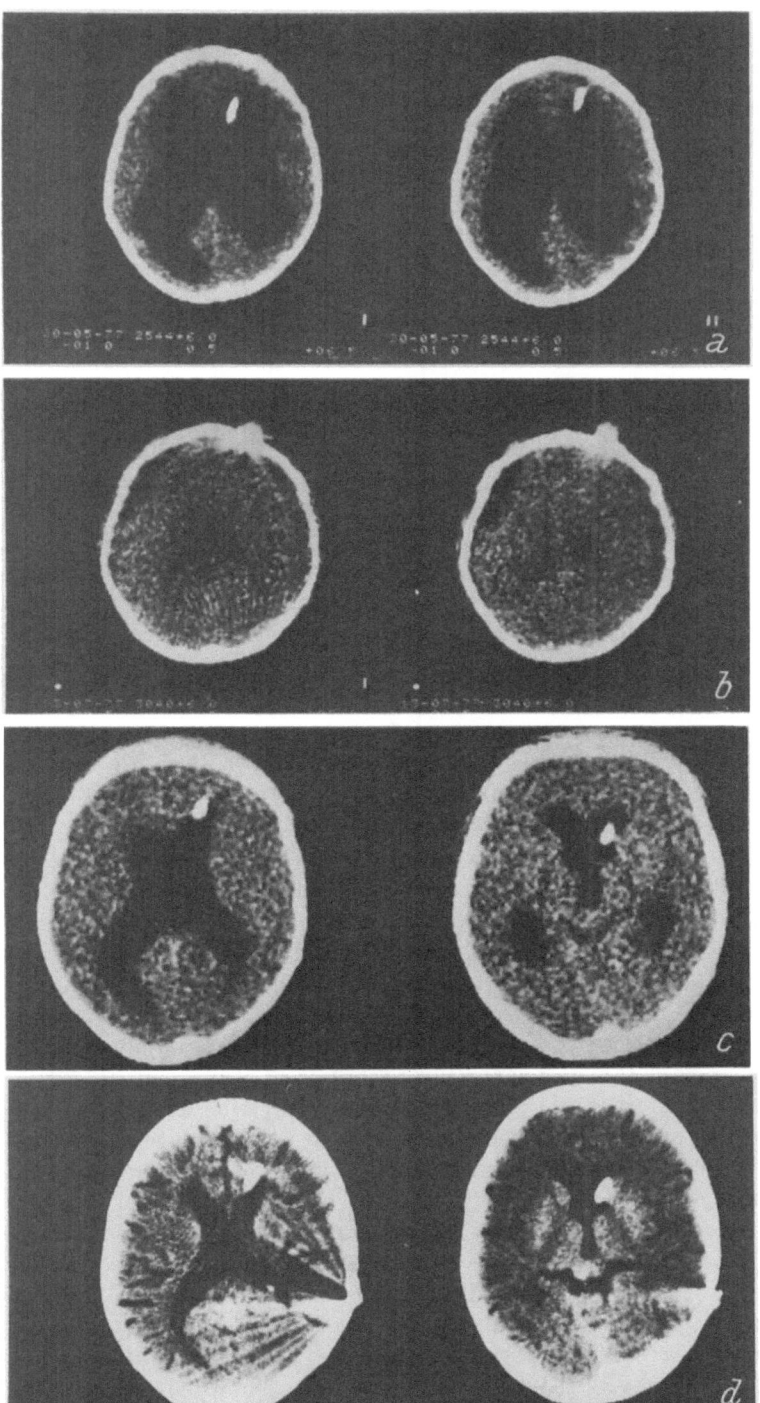

Fig. 9. CCT-follow-up study. (a) Extreme hydrocephalus due to aqueduct stenosis. (b) Few weeks after insertion of a medium pressure peritoneal shunt: subdural effusions. (c) One year later: shunt occlusion resulting in ventricular dilatation, the subdural effusions have disappeared. (d) Normalisation of ventricular size after insertion of a high-pressure atrial shunt

shunt obstruction secondary to *small ventricles* the indication for craniotomy was quite different. Epstein suggested temporal craniectomy on the side of the ventricular catheter because since Kaufman (1973) it has been known that the drained ventricle tends to be much smaller. Furthermore laboratory investigation (Hochwald 1973) suggested that temporal craniotomy would encourage an ipsilateral ventricle to dilate, which in turn would protect against further catheter obstruction. Later Holness (1979) has reported his results using subtemporal decompression for the *slit ventricle* syndrome with repeated ventricular catheter occlusion in 22 cases: the frequency of hospitalization for shunt revision was greatly reduced although in several cases additional interventions were needed; in 6 cases upper end revisions and in 4 cases insertion of antisiphon devices. In Walsh's (1979) series 7 children underwent subtemporal craniectomy. These patients improved having either no further shunt malfunction or malfunctions with symptoms of less severity. 3 patients however continued with persistent shunt obstructions, they and one other patient received a new valve with higher resistance and improved. In 1978 Salmon reported 4 cases with collapsed ventricles. They were treated by adding a higher pressure valve to the diversionary system: the ventricles enlarged and they became asymptomatic. Following the concept of elective shunt revision (Becker and Nulsen 1968). Salmon (1979) presented 43 cases in whome electively on the occasion of shunt lengthening a higher pressure valve was added. None of these patients developed slit like ventricles.

Hoffman (1976) reported cerebellar herniation in cases with *cerebrocranial disproportion* following lumboperitoneal shunts. He treated these cases successfully with a posterior fossa decompression. Tonsillar herniation following the shunting procedure seems to be a special sequel to lumboperitoneal shunting.

Generally, in most clinical reports (Hemmer 1966, Illingworth 1970, Samuelson 1972, McCullough 1974, Portnoy 1973) the surgical evacuation of the *subdural haematoma* or *hygroma* is advised. Indeed in some cases operative intervention cannot be avoided. In most cases, however, an expectant attitude with adequate controls is justified. Our experience with 12 untreated subdural lesions in valve patients, seems to confirm this regime (Faulhauer 1978). Emery (1965) in the above mentioned neuropathological study, has described chronic subdural haematomas which did not cause compression of the underlying brain. In addition, he has described in many cases augmentation of the subdural connective tissue and a thickening of the arachnoid. He characterized these structures as space fillers.

Our cases with subdural callus would not have profited from burr hole drainage. which was done by Illingworth (1970) and Samuelson (1972) in most of their cases. The latter were adults, whereas our patients were children between two and twelve years of age. Only the case of Hemmer (1966) described as haematoma was similar to ours. Hemmer, Illingworth and Samuelson have occluded or removed the CSF shunt at the same time. Illingworth needed ventricular drainage in four cases. All our treated patients needed external ventricular drainage (Faulhauer 1978).

In 1974 Portnoy suggested simultaneous drainage of the ventricles and subdural space, whereby the outflow of CSF is regulated by a differential pressure valve. In our experience, however, those subdural effusions which can be drained that way, are mostly asymptomatic and disappear whenever additional space is needed.

The poor results of Illingworth and Samuelson and also our depressing experiences with surgically treated subdural lesions in valve patients justify in most cases an expectant attitude after careful consideration of risks.

V. Prevention of Overdrainage

1. The Role of Valvular Closing Pressure in the Origin of Overdrainage

A detailed discussion about pressure/flow characteristics of valves and their influence on proper or excessive drainage of hydrocephalus is beyond the scope of this chapter. For many years it has been a common practice to use low pressure slit valves in the treatment of newborn hydrocephalus (McNab 1959, Pertuiset 1971, Anderson 1966, Salmon 1979). It was argued, that newborn hydrocephalus is a "low pressure hydrocephalus". By application of physical principles it has been shown, that the larger the ventricular size, the lower is the level to which intraventricular pressure must be reduced in order to achieve effective shunting with reduction of ventricular size (Hakim 1972, Early 1976). It was also proposed to use low pressure valves in order to avoid peritoneal shunt obstruction (Raimondi 1975). Only few authors have reported about overdrainage symptoms and have related them to low pressure valves: Anderson (1966) and Kloss (1968) have seen the relationship between low pressure valves and craniostenosis and changed over to medium pressure valves. Even with the use of medium pressure valves however, Roberts (1970) observed craniostenosis. Collapsed or slit ventricles cephalocranial disproportion has also been reported as result of low pressure systems or extracranial drainage without valvular resistance (Salmon 1978, Holness 1979, Hoffman 1976). Schmitz (1979) observed 88 persistent overdrainage signs (microcrania, slit ventricles, intolerance to minimal pressure rises and subdural haematoma) in 49 cases out of 400 shunted patients. He determined the opening pressure of those valves which were thought to be responsible for overdrainage: over 60% had low pressure valves, almost 80% low or medium pressure valves and only 20% of the hyperdrained hydrocephalic patients had high pressure valves.

Low resistance valves seem to favour hyperdrainage symptoms, high pressure valves cannot prevent them in all cases. As we have seen siphon effect and negative pressure valves in the right atrium may easily overcome the closing pressure of a high pressure valve.

2. Specially Designed Valves and Devices for Preventing Post-Shunt Overdrainage

In 1973 Portnoy presented the *antisiphon device*, which was added to conventional diverting systems in order to reduce the hazard of negative intraventricular pressure when the patient is sitting or standing. He and McCullough (1974) however noted that subdural haematoma cannot always be

18 K. Faulhauer:

prevented with these units. It is Portnoy's conviction, that most chronic subdural haematomas occur at the time of valve placement because of the cerebral mantle collapse. He, therefore, also in 1973, adviced the additional use of *percutaneously reversible occlusion valves*.

This valve is closed after shunt insertion and opened percutaneously 3 or 4 days later, when the cerebral mantle is reexpanded. In a personal communica-

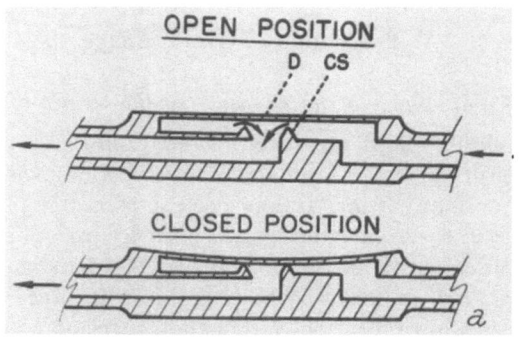

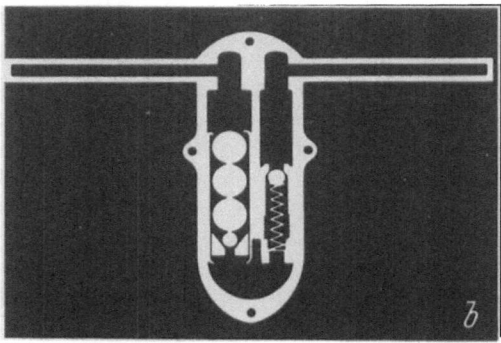

Fig. 10. Diagrams of the antisiphon device (a) and the Cordis horizontal-vertical lumboperitoneal shunt system

tion Portnoy (1980) mentioned that since he has been using the ASD over 7 years he has not had a patient with symptoms related to overdrainage.

Salah (1978) recently presented his experience with 38 cases who received valve combinations including the antisiphon device. Minor problems due to overdrainage occurred in only two cases: asymptomatic bilateral effusions and low pressure headaches.

Jones in 1978 published his experiences with antisiphon devices in 111 patients. 34 patients had an antisiphon device incorporated in a valve as primary procedure. In this group there was only one case with subdural effusion. In 77 cases the antisiphon device was added to a conventional high or medium pressure valve. In these cases the author noted a great number of hypotensive and hypertensive complications. He concluded therefore that it is preferable to use antisiphon devices initially to avoid symptoms and signs associated with sudden change in pressure.

Yamada (1979) constructed an *antisiphon ball valve*, which has a silicone cylinder and a movable enclosed stainless steel ball. The valve closes in the

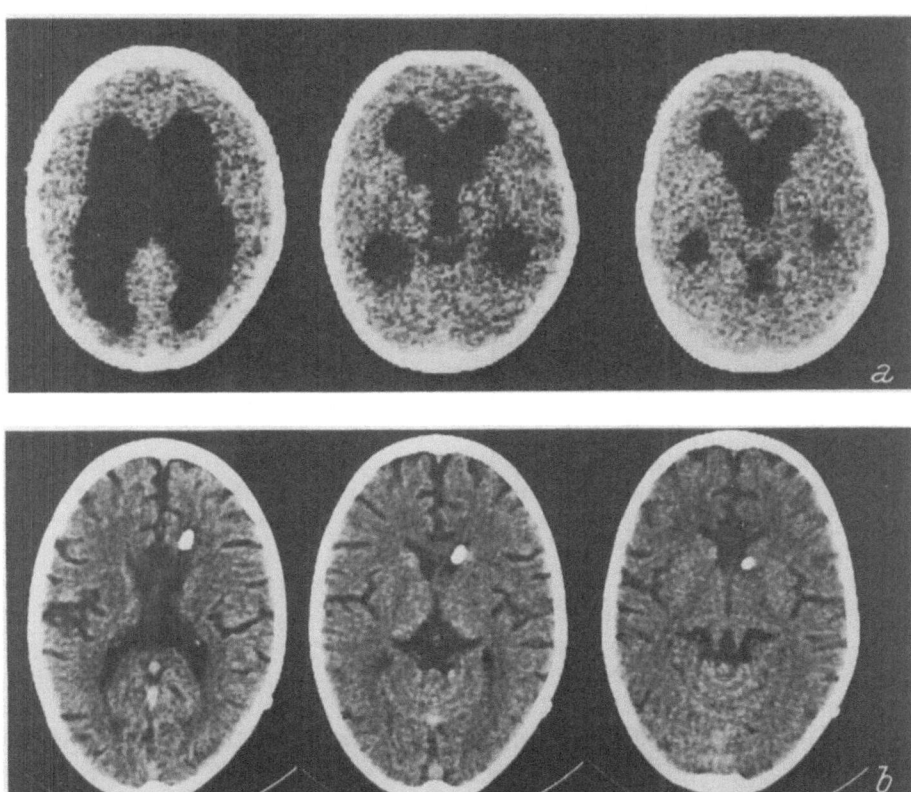

Fig. 11. (a) CCT of a large hydrocephalus secondary to aqueduct stenosis. (b) Normalisation of ventricular size after insertion of a ventriculo-peritoneal shunt with antisiphon device

vertical position and is released in the horizontal position. The author used this device together with ventriculoperitoneal shunts in 45 cases and found it useful to prevent post-shunt overdrainage syndromes.

The same principle is applied in the *Cordis horizontalvertical lumbar-peritoneal valve system*. It is a combination of a differential pressure ball valve and a gravity occlusion device. To the best of the author's knowledge clinical experience has not yet been published.

VI. Future Perspectives

The general discontent with available possibilities in the treatment of hydrocephalus has not only created a vast diversification of different shunting systems, it has also promoted a great number of new approaches and a search for new concepts. There are several trials to inhibit CSF production on a pharmacological basis, *e.g.* by medication with acetazolamide (Smith 1974) and isorbide (Lorber 1973) or by radionecrosis of the choroid plexus (Weiss 1972).

With special reference to the overdrainage syndrome Epstein has suggested several quite unconventional therapeutic measures: on the basis of Hochwald's (1972) experimentally presumed transventricular CSF absorption as the alternate pathway he tried to convert the progressive in arrested hydrocephalus by means of the *volume control shunt* (1973) and later by *head wrapping* (1973) in small infants. Epstein's controversial suggestions were abandoned however when in 1972 Eisenberg showed, that in Kaolin induced feline hydrocephalus, compensation occurred through the dilating central canal.

In the discussion about the ideal extracranial CSF diversion several authors have proposed *valves with variable closing pressure* in order to adjust the valvular function according to the actual need. Hakim (1974) has announced such a valve. Hildebrandt (1976) has outlined a variable pressure valve with transcutaneous pressure recording and adjustment. Sahar (1979) has reported an animal experiments with valves, where closing pressure can be changed externally by a magnetic field.

A *self-adjusting pressure valve* was designed many years ago by Hakim in which the closing pressure was continuously adjusted in inverse proportion to the subdural stress exerted on a subdural balloon. Unfortunately this valve was never produced.

In order to improve CSF absorption the implantation of omentum in the ventricular CSF space was carried out successfully in animal experiments (Yaşargil 1974). After very careful evaluation in animal experiments Levander *et al.* (1978) successfully treated patients with communicating hydrocephalus by performing lumboomental shunts.

Al Sharif *et al.* (1978) reported on a series of patients with infantile progressive hydrocephalus—communicating or non-communicating—which had been treated with reasonably good results by introducing a pedicled pericranial flap into the ventricle.

Both Levander's lumbo-omental shunt and Al Sharif's pericranial flap methods seem to be promising developments which should be continued and, if the initial good results are reproducible, introduced into neurosurgical routine.

VII. Conclusions

1. Extracranial CSF diversions often result in acute or chronic overdrainage syndromes.

2. Acute decompression and low pressure headaches are sometimes very troublesome but actually easy to handle.

3. Most significant however is the excessive reduction of CSF volume leading to slit ventricles, microcrania and loss of the adaptive mechanisms for intracranial pressure elevations.

4. Subdural effusions and haematomas are probably much more frequent

than generally accepted. In most cases they are "space-filling" rather than space-occupying.

5. Treatment of "subdural haematoma" therefore only is indicated when clinical findings suggest cerebral compression, which means real space-occupation. In most cases only regular consecutive controls are necessary.

6. In cases of repeated ventricular catheter occlusion due to slit ventricles the replacement of valves of too low a pressure by valves with higher opening pressure will be of great value. When shunt obstruction results in cerebral decompensation due to intolerance of pressure elevations in cases with slit ventricles, subtemporal decompression may be the only measure to save the patient's life.

7. Overdrainage cannot be avoided completely but the use of higher pressure valves will certainly reduce the incidence of overdrainage signs. There is evidence, that the addition of the antisiphon device will reduce the danger of negative intracranial pressure, when the patient is in erect position.

8. The tendency for all differential pressure valves to overdrain the CSF space has promoted the sample for new therapeutic concepts like Levander's lumboomental shunt and Al Sharif's pericranial flap operation, and also for better shunting systems.

References

Al Sharif, H., Abdoul-Dahb, Y. W., Abdel-Hafez, M. S., Ghaly, A. F., Hussein, A., 1978: The pericranium flap operation. A new operation for the treatment of progressive infantile hydrocephalus. Acta neurochir. (Wien) *41*, 335—347.

Anderson, F. M., 1952: Subdural hematoma, a complication of operation for hydrocephalus. Pediatrics *10*, 11—18.

Anderson, H., 1966: Craniosynostosis as a complication after operation for hydrocephalus. Acta Paediat. Scand. *55*, 192—196.

Becker, D. P., Nulsen, F. E., 1968: Control of hydrocephalus by valve-regulated venous shunt: avoidance of complications in prolonged shunt maintenance. J. Neurosurg. *28*, 215—225.

Early, C. B., Fink, L. H., 1976: Some fundamental applications of the law of La Place in neurosurgery. Surg. Neurol. *6*, 185—189.

Eisenberg, H. M., McLennan, J. E., Welch, K., 1974: Ventricular perfusion in cats with kaolin-induced hydrocephalus. J. Neurosurg. *41*, 20—28.

Emery, J. L., 1965: Intracranial effects of longstanding decompression of the brain in children with hydrocephalus and meningomyelocele. Develop. Med. Child Neurol. *7*, 302—309.

Epstein, F., 1973: A volume control system for the treatment of hydrocephalus: laboratory and clinical experience. J. Neurosurg. *38*, 282—287.

— 1973: Neonatal hydrocephalus treated by head wrapping. The Lancet No. 7804, 634—636.

— 1974: Subtemporal craniectomy for recurrent shunt obstruction secondary to small ventricles. J. Neurosurg. *41*, 29—31.

— 1975: Letter to the editor. J. Neurosurg. *42*, 116.

— 1977: Role of computerized axial tomography in diagnosis, treatment and follow-up of hydrocephalus. Child's Brain *3*, 91—100.

Faulhauer, K., Kremer, G., Lehmann, H., 1975: Untersuchungen über die Häufigkeit und klinische Bedeutung des ventilunabhängigen, zum Stillstand gekommenen Hydrozephalus. Klin. Pädiat. *187*, 432—442.

— Schmitz, P., 1978: Overdrainage phenomena in shunt treated hydrocephalus. Acta neurochir. (Wien) *45*, 89—101.

Forrest, D. M., Cooper, D. G. W., 1968: Complications of ventriculo-atrial shunts. A review of 455 cases. J. Neurosurg. *29*, 506—512.

Fox, J. L., 1973: Cerebrospinal fluid shunts: An experimental evaluation of flow rates and pressure values in the anti-siphon valve. Surg. Neurol. *1*, 299—302.

Griscom, N. T., Oh, K. S., 1970: The contracting skull. Inward growth of the inner table as a physiologic response to diminution of intracranial content in children. Amer. J. Roentgenol. *110*, 106—110.

Guidetti, B., 1976: Hydrocephalus in infancy and childhood. Child's Brain *2*, 209—225.

Hakim, S., 1972: Biomechanics of hydrocephalus, in cisternography and hydrocephalus (Harbert, H. C., ed.). Springfield, Ill.: Ch. C Thomas.

— 1974: Personal communication.

— Venegas, J. G.: The need for a self-adjusting pressure valve in the treatment of hydrocephalus. Paper distributed by the Cordis Company.

Harbert, J., 1974: Quantitation of cerebrospinal fluid shunt flow. Radiology *112*, 379—387.

Hayden, P. W., Rudd, T. G., Ditzmang, D., Shurtleff, D. B., 1974: Evaluation of surgically treated hydrocephalus by radionuclide clearance studies of the cerebrospinal fluid shunts. 18th Annual Meeting of the Society for Research into Hydrocephalus and Spina Bifida. Göteborg.

Hemmer, R., 1966: Subdurales Hämatom als Begleiterscheinung des ventrikuloaurikulären Shunts. Neurochirurgica *9*, 114—118.

— 1977: Surgical treatment of hydrocephalus: Complications, mortality, developmental prospects. Z. Kinderchir. *22*, 443—452.

Hildebrandt, J. J., Plitz, W., Herrmann, H. D., 1976: Erfindungsmeldung.

Hochwald, G. M., Epstein, F., Malhan, C., Ransohoff, J., 1973: The relationship of compensated to decompensated hydrocephalus in the cat. J. Neurosurg. *39*, 694—697.

— Lux, W. E., Sahar, A., Ransohoff, J., 1972: Experimental hydrocephalus. Changes in cerebrospinal fluid dynamics as a function of time. Arch. Neurol. *26*, 120—129.

Hoffman, H. J., 1976: Cephalocranial disproportion. Child's Brain *2*, 167—176.

Holness, R. O., Hoffman, H. J., Hendrick, E. B., 1979: Subtemporal decompression for the slit-ventricle syndrome after shunting in hydrocephalic children. Child's Brain *5*, 137—144.

Holtzer, G. J., Lange, S. A., de, 1973: Shunt independent arrest of hydrocephalus. J. Neurosurg. *39*, 698—701.

Illingworth, R. D., 1970: Subdural hematoma after the treatment of chronic hydrocephalus by ventriculocaval shunts. J. Neurol. Neurosurg. Psychiat. *33*, 95—99.

Ito, M., Tsugane, R., Ohya, M., Bun, M., Sato, O., 1979: Slit-like ventricle after the shunt operation for hydrocephalus. Child's Brain *5*, 580.

Jackson, I. J., Snodgrass, S. R., 1955: Peritoneal shunts in the treatment of hydrocephalus and increased intracranial pressure. J. Neurosurg. *12*, 216—222.

Jones, R., 1979: Experience with anti-siphon devices at the Prince of Wales Children's Hospital. Child's Brain *5*, 555.

Kaufman, B., Weiss, M. H., Young, H. F., Nulsen, F. E., 1973: Effects of prolonged cerebrospinal fluid shunting on the skull and brain. J. Neurosurg. *38*, 288—297.

Keucher, T. R., Mealey, Jr., J., 1979: Long-term results after ventriculoatrial and ventriculoperitoneal shunting for infantile hydrocephalus. J. Neurosurg. *50*, 179—186.

Kirch, E., 1977: Klinische Erfahrungen mit der Ventrikulozisternostomie nach Torkildsen. Dissertation, Homburg/Saar.

Kloss, J. L., 1968: Craniosynostosis secondary to ventriculoatrial shunt. Amer. J. Dis. Child. *116*, 315—317.

Levander, B., Åsard, P.-E., 1978: Lumbo-omental shunt for drainage of cerebrospinal fluid. — An experimental study in dogs. I.: The transport of cerebrospinal fluid from the lumbar subarachnoid space, studied by [169]Yb-DTPA and a gamma camera. Acta neurochir. (Wien) *43*, 1—11.

Levander, B., Bergvall, U., Wennerstrand, J., Åsard, P.-E., 1974: Omental transposition for drainage of cerebrospinal fluid. The Lancet No. *7883*, 776—777, September 28, 1974.
— — — — 1975: Omental transposition for drainage of cerebrospinal fluid in man. The Lancet No. 7937, 702—703, October 11, 1975.
— Zwetnow, N. N., 1978: Bulk flow of cerebrospinal fluid through a lumbo-omental graft in the dog. Acta neurochir. (Wien) *41*, 147—156.
— Granberg, P. O., Hindmarsh, T., 1978: Lumbo-omental shunt for drainage of cerebrospinal fluid in hydrocephalus. Acta neurochir. (Wien) *44*, 1—9.
Lorber, J., 1973: Isosorbide in the medical treatment of infantile hydrocephalus. J. Neurosurg. *39*, 702—711.

Meese, W., Lanksch, W., Wende, S., 1976: Diagnosis and postoperative follow-up studies of infantile hydrocephalus using computerized tomography. In: Cranial computerized tomography by (Lanksch, W., Kazner, E., eds.). Berlin-Heidelberg-New York: Springer.
McCullough, D. C., Fox, J. L., 1974: Negative intracranial pressure hydrocephalus in adults with shunts and its relationship to the production of subdural hematoma. J. Neurosurg. *40*, 372—375.
McNab, G. H., 1959: The Spitz-Holter valve. J. Neurol. Neurosurg. Psychiat. *22*, 82—83.
Moseley, J., 1978: CT Scanning in the management of patients after ventricular shunting. Abstract in: XI. Symposium Neuroradiologicum, Wiesbaden.
Nulsen, F. E., Spitz, E. B., 1952: Treatment of hydrocephalus by direct shunt from ventricle to jugular vein. Surg. Forum *2*, 399.
Pertuiset, B., 1971: Therapy of congenital hydrocephalus in infancy. Progr. neurol. Surg. *4*, 289—328.
Portnoy, H. D., 1980: Personal communication.
— Croissant, P. D., 1974: Combined drainage of ventricular and subdural fluid. Surg. Neurol. *2*, 41—42:
— Schulte, R. R., Fox, J. L., Croissant, P. D., Tripp, L., 1973: Anti-siphon and reversible occlusion valves for shunting in hydrocephalus and preventing post-shunt subdural hematomas. J. Neurosurg. *38*, 729—738.
Raimondi, A. J., 1975: Personal communication.
— Robinson, J. S., Kuwamura, K., 1977: Complications of ventriculoperitoneal shunting and a critical comparison of the three-piece and one-piece systems. Child's Brain *3*, 321—342.

Rayport, M., Reiss, J., 1969: Hydrodynamic properties of certain shunt assemblies for the treatment of hydrocephalus. J. Neurosurg. *30*, 455—467.

Roberts, J. R., Rickham, P. P., 1970: Craniostenosis following holter valve operation. Develop. Med. Child Neurol. Suppl. *22*, 145—149.

Sahar, A., Ron, S., Levy, I., 1979: Variable pressure valve for hydrocephalus shunt systems. Child's Brain *5*, 555.

Salah, S., Sunder-Plassmann, M., Zaunbauer, F., Koos, W., 1978: The use of the anti-siphon valve in prevention of functional complications in shunting system. Advances in Neurosurgery, Vol. *6* (Wüllenweber, R., ed.), pp. 42—44. Berlin-Heidelberg-New York: Springer.

Salmon, J. H., 1978: The collapsed ventricle: management and prevention. Surg. Neurol. *9*, 349—352.
— 1979: Management of the slit-like ventricle. Child's Brain *5*, 557.

Samuelson, S., Long, D. M., Chou, S. N., 1972: Subdural hematoma as a complication of shunting procedures for normal pressure hydrocephalus. J. Neurosurg. *37*, 548—552.

Scarff, J. E., 1963: Treatment of hydrocephalus. An historical and critical review of methods and results. J. Neurol. Neurosurg. Psychiat. *26*, 1—48.

Shurtleff, D. B., Kronmal, R., Foltz, E. L., 1975: Follow-up comparison of hydrocephalus with and without myelomeningocele. J. Neurosurg. *42*, 61—68.
Smith, R. V., Roberts, P. A., Fisher, R. G., 1974: Alteration of cerebrospinal fluid production in the dog. Surg. Neurol. *2*, 267—269.

Schmitz, P., 1979: Klinische Folgen der exzessiven Liquordrainage bei extrakraniellen Liquorshunts. Dissertation, Homburg/Saar.

Steinbok, P., Thompson, G. B., 1976: Complications of ventriculo-vascular shunts: Computer analysis of etiological factors. Surg. Neurol. 5, 31—35.

Venes, J. L., 1978: Computerized axial tomography in the management of the child with shunted hydrocephalus. Z. Kinderchir. 25, 330—335.

Villani, R., Gaini, S. M., Giovanelli, M., Tomei, G., Zavanone, M., 1976: Skull modifications after CSF-shunt for infantile hydrocephalus. 20th Annual Meeting of the Society for Research into hydrocephalus and spina bifida. Bern.

Walsh, J. W., 1979: Subtemporal decompression and elevation of shunt valve pressure in the management of transient shunt obstruction from slit ventricles. Child's Brain 5, 556.

Weiss, M. H., Nulsen, F. E., Kaufmann, B., 1972: Selective radionecrosis of the choroid plexus for control of experimental hydrocephalus. J. Neurosurg. 36, 270—275.

Yamada, H., Tajima, M., Nagaya, M., 1975: Effect of respiratory movement on cerebrospinal fluid dynamics in hydrocephalic infants with shunts. J. Neurosurg. 42, 194—200.

— Funakoshi, T., Ando, T., Sakai, N., Sakata, K., 1979: Clinical studies on prevention of overdrainage syndrome after ventriculoperitoneal shunt by use of an antisiphon ball valve. Child's Brain 5, 556.

Yamada, S., Ducker, T. B., Perot, P. L., 1975: Dynamic changes of cerebrospinal fluid in upright and recumbent shunted experimental animals. Child's Brain 1, 187—192.

Yaşargil, M. G., Yonekawa, Y., Denton, J., Proth, D., Benes, I., 1974: Experimental intracranial transplantation of autogenic omentum majus. J. Neurosurg. 39, 213—217.

Intravascular Occlusion of Saccular Aneurysms of the Cerebral Arteries by Means of a Detachable Balloon Catheter

A. P. Romodanov and V. I. Shcheglov

Kiev Research Institute of Neurosurgery, Kiev (USSR)

With 12 Figures

Contents

I. Introduction

Among the numerous methods of treatment of saccular arterial cerebral aneurysms particular attention has been recently focused on intravascular intervention using detachable balloon catheters. The last decade was marked by active development, perfection and successful practical application of this technique (Serbinenko 1971, 1974 a, b; Zubkov 1974, 1979; Romodanov *et al.* 1975, 1979 a, b; Debrun *et al.* 1975, 1978; Zozulia, Shcheglov 1976; Shcheglov 1976, 1979; Lazarev, Lysachev 1978; Laitinen *et al.* 1978; DiTullio *et al.* 1978; Taki *et al.* 1979).

In 1930 Brooks having advanced an original intravascular approach to the treatment of some cerebrovascular diseases, inserted a muscle strip into the carotid artery to embolize a carotid cavernous fistula.

Brooks' concept was further developed by Luessenhop *et al.* (1960) who introduced the term "surgical embolization" and made trials to embolize arteriovenous malformations with plastic balls.

The idea of using a detachable balloon catheter ("angioblockader") for temporary or permanent occlusion of major veins and arteries was advanced by Misiuk (1960) but at that time his device did not pass into clinical practice.

Rothenberg *et al.* (1962) invented a device for endovascular interventions consisting of syringe, cardiac catheter and a metal carrier with a balloon and introduced the term "angiotactic surgery" for intravascular operations. After successful animal experimentation they suggested clinical application of the device primarily for the management of certain saccular aneurysms. Fogarty *et al.* (1963) recommended the employment of a non-detachable balloon catheter for removal of thrombi and emboli from major vessels. It proved possible by means of this catheter and the like to obliterate successfully intracranial aneurysms together with their parent vessels (Kessler, Wholey 1970; Wholey *et al.* 1972).

Of major importance for the further development of intravascular interventions was the contribution of Luessenhop and Velasquez (1964) and Luessenhop (1978). They were the first to introduce a balloon catheter into the supraclinoid portion of the carotid artery and to prove the feasibility of occluding the orifice of a supraclinoid aneurysm with an inflatable silicone balloon. They also made the important observation that catheterization of the brain vessels induced no arterial spasm. However, wide clinical use of their balloon catheter technique met with difficulties because intravascular manoeuvering was flow-directed and, thus, uncontrollable.

Alksne (1968), Yodh *et al.* (1968) tried to improve the delivery of the balloon catheter to the target brain vessels by means of an electromagnetic system. At present wider clinical application of this method is fraught with technical difficulties.

A qualitatively new stage and perspective of current development of intravascular surgery is connected with the name of Serbinenko who developed and applied clinically the method of catheterization and artificial occlusion of the brain vessels by means of different microballoon catheters including the detachable balloon catheter (Serbinenko 1971, 1972, 1974 a, b). Serbinenko's invention solved the problem of catheterization of the main brain arteries and their large branches. Of particular value in Serbinenko's method is the possibility of controllable delivery of the balloon catheter to the brain vessels. The balloon catheter may be selectively placed at the planned site of the artery and if necessary removed from the vessel. The construction allows detachment the catheter from the balloon, thus, permitting permanent occlusion of an artery, aneurysm etc. The way thus proved open for fundamentally new operations on the brain vessels. Particularly tempting was Serbinenko's comment about the possibility of performing reconstructive operations for saccular aneurysms. This innovation allowed obliteration of the aneurysm by a detachable balloon preserving the patency and functional validity of the parent vessel. This operation was first performed by Serbinenko in 1973 (Serbinenko 1974). The experience of Serbinenko demonstrated favourable results in the treatment of patients with carotid-cavernous fistulas, arteriovenous malformations and some saccular cerebral aneurysms. This attracted considerable neurosurgical interest towards intravascular operations.

Zubkov (1973, 1979) operated on 24 patients with the purpose of occluding cerebral saccular aneurysms by means of a detachable balloon catheter. Successful occlusion was, however, performed only in 14 patients. Reconstructive surgery was performed in 9 of these patients.

At the Kiev Research Institute of Neurosurgery reconstructive detachable balloon catheter surgery was initiated in 1974 for different cerebral vascular lesions including two patients with saccular aneurysms. The patency and function of the aneurysm-bearing vessel were preserved in these instances (Romodanov et al. 1975, 1979; Zozulia and Shcheglov 1976; Shcheglov 1976). Encouraged by this success these authors spared no effort in further development of endovascular treatment of intracranial saccular aneurysms (Romodanov and Shcheglov 1979; Shcheglov 1979).

Debrun and his associates (1975, 1978) contributed much to the development of balloon catheter interventions. Their experimental and clinical work and cautious approach to establishing the indications for these operations and their critical attitude to the results obtained should not be underestimated. These workers, however, suggest that the detachable balloon technique seems restricted to a very limited number of saccular aneurysm cases, in particular, anterior communicating artery aneurysms should not be treated by this method. Debrun et al. (1978) obtained favourable results in 7 of 14 patients operated on for intracranial aneurysms of the carotid siphon. Reconstructive surgery was performed in 5 patients.

Zlotnik et al. (1978) reported occlusion of saccular supraclinoid carotid aneurysms in 6 patients by the Serbinenko technique. Lazarev et al. (1978) analysed their 7-year experience with the treatment of saccular arterial cerebral aneurysms by the Serbinenko detachable balloon catheter. Reconstructive surgery was performed in 4 of their 25 patients with aneurysms of the intracranial portion of the carotid artery. In the remaining cases carotid occlusion was performed at the aneurysm orifice level (14 cases) and at the C-1 vertebra level (7 cases).

Recently, several new types of detachable balloon catheters have been developed and used experimentally (Laitinen, Servo 1978; DiTullio et al. 1978) or both experimentally and clinically (Taki et al. 1978). An essentially new method of releasing the catheter from the balloon was proposed by Taki et al. (1979). To prevent breaks and kinkings of the catheter during its insertion into the brain vessels these authors protect the catheter with a silicone tube. The balloon catheter is flexible and can easily be inserted into the branches of the middle, posterior or anterior cerebral arteries. Firm ties prevent accidental release of the balloon. They reported successful occlusion in a patient with a saccular middle cerebral artery aneurysm but only further clinical experience may reveal the advantages of this newly developed balloon catheter.

This brief review of the literature is evidence of the growing interest in the fundamentally new intravascular reconstructive operations by means of the releasable balloon catheters and the reality of successful management of saccular arterial cerebral aneurysms by this method.

II. Making and Construction of the Detachable Balloon Catheter

We have used different balloon catheters beginning in 1974 for the occlusion of saccular arterial cerebral aneurysms including the detachable Serbinenko catheter and consider that in the latter balloon-to-catheter ties are very convenient allowing union over a varying range, from easily releasable to rigid. In the course of our work we have made modifications in the construction of the Serbinenko balloon catheter, particularly with the purpose of management of small (under 0.6-0.8 cm in diameter) saccular arterial cerebral aneurysms. Based on the Serbinenko technique we invented in 1978 (coauthors S. A. Romodanov and A. G. Savenko) a balloon catheter ("occluding device") designed specially for the management of saccular aneurysms of the cerebral arteries.

The balloon is made by dipping a cylindrical metal or plastic mould (from 0.2 to 1.4 mm in diameter) into pure latex. The thickness of the balloon wall depends on the viscous properties of latex and the speed of removal of the mould from the latex as well as on the number of immersions of the mould in the latex mass. The balloon wall thickness may vary from 0.1 to 0.15 mm. The latex mass is allowed to dry on the mould for 10-20 minutes at room temperature. The mould with the balloon on it are then immersed in talcum, dried at room temperature for 2-3 hours. The balloon is then delicately and cautiously slipped off the mould. Length of the prepared balloon: from 3-8 mm to 2-3 cm; external diamter: 0.6-1.8 mm. On inflation by air or fluid the balloon diameter increases 6-8 times (Fig. 1). The tail of the balloon is transformed into a sphincter by putting 2-3 thin latex rings on it. The rings are fastened to the balloon by latex. The balloon with the sphincter on its tail is now a single device. The sphincter stretches when the balloon is inflated. A radiopaque marker (usually silver wire, 2-3 mm long and 0.3-0.4 mm thick) is placed inside the head of the balloon and fixed by monofiber. This marker allows observation of the the course of the balloon during the entire procedure.

A soft polyethylene tube (diameter: 0.5-0.7-1.0 mm) of high tensile properties and strength is used as a catheter. The end of the catheter which is to be introduced into the tail of the balloon, has a conical shape with thickening of the tip. The tip of the catheter is thickened by heating and covering with several latex layers. The thickening may be of various forms and sizes. The balloon with the sphincter on its tail plus catheter are thus an integral balloon catheter device. The balloon is held on the catheter so that the former is not released accidentally into the blood stream and, if necessary, can be purposefully detached from the catheter or returned to the puncture needle. This system of union allowing alteration of the strength of the sphincter, form and size of thickening, guarantees high mobility of the balloon in relation to the catheter

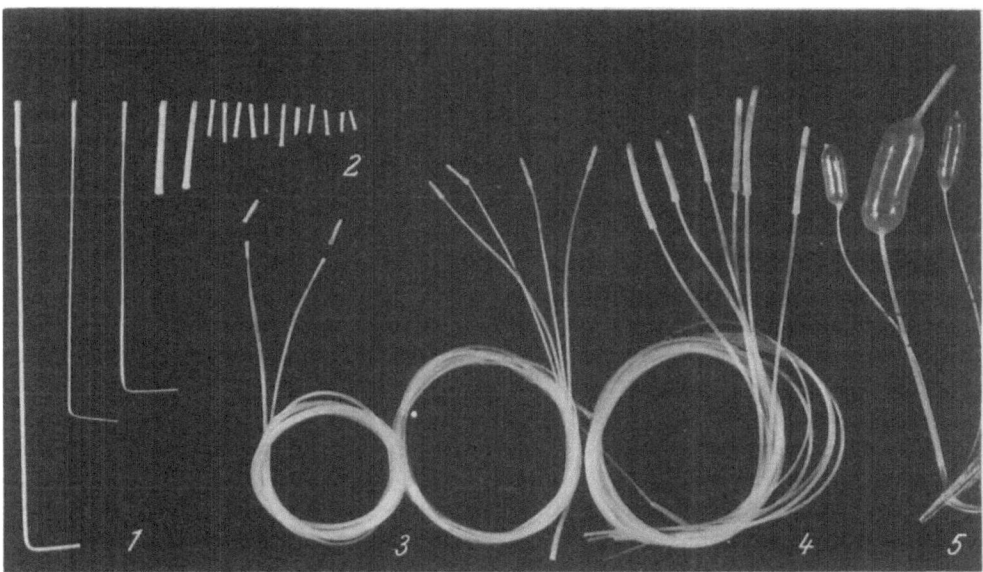

Fig. 1. Balloons and balloon catheters (natural sizes). *1* Balloons on mould; *2* Balloons removed from mould; *3* Balloons and catheters ready for union; *4* Balloon catheters for occlusion of saccular aneurysms; *5* Inflated balloons

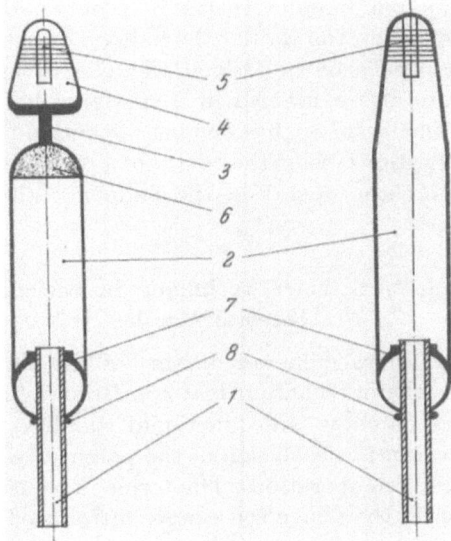

Fig. 2. Two types of balloon catheters. *1* Catheter; *2* Balloon; *3* Elastic bridge; *4* Anterior mobile part of balloon; *5* Silver mark; *6* Radiopaque tantalum dust; *7* Sphincter; *8* Silver ring

and secure fixation of the balloon on the catheter during catheterization of the brain arteries. The balloon may be easily deliberately detached after being filled with a radiopaque substance or a quickly hardening biologically inert polymer (silicone). The rounded form and smooth surface of the balloon promote its introduction into the major arteries, their large branches and into the aneurysmal cavity. A similar form of the tail of the balloon favours removal of the balloon in the reverse direction and its return into the lumen of the needle, *e.g.* when it is necessary to replace one balloon catheter by another in the course of the operation or when the situation makes it mandatory to discontinue the operation. For better orientation of the neurosurgeon concerning the position of the balloon in the aneurysm, particularly in the small aneurysm, we frequently place a radiopaque marker (miniature silver ring) near the sphincter. This marker is fastened only to the catheter and when the latter is released from the balloon, the marker is removed from the circulation together with the catheter.

For occlusion of saccular arterial cerebral aneurysms we make also another special type of detachable balloon catheter. An elastic bridge is mounted on the balloon. One end of this bridge is rigidly connected with the main inflatable part of the balloon, the other with the working radiopaque part of the balloon (Fig. 2). This increases significantly the manoeuverability of the balloon. Fluctuations and turns of the radiopaque working part of the balloon are of help in evaluating the site where linear blood flow becomes turbulent at the level of the aneurysmal orifice. Besides the main detachable balloon catheter we also use an auxiliary nondetachable balloon catheter. It differs from the former that the tail of the balloon at the sphincter level is additionally fastened to the catheter by monofiber. The prepared balloon catheter is maximally filled with air to establish possible defects in the wall of the balloon or catheter, to evaluate the proportion of different parts of the balloon, the reliability of balloon-to-catheter ties. The balloons are also examined in a specially designed artificial elastic transparent plastic aneurysm so that one may evaluate the "behaviour" of the balloon in similar conditions inside the cavity of a real aneurysm or in the artery lumen. Directly before the operation the balloon catheters are sterilized in alcohol for 10 minutes.

III. Detachable Balloon Catheter Technique in Saccular Aneurysms of the Cerebral Arteries

The management of saccular aneurysms of the cerebral arteries by the detachable balloon catheter technique may consist of occlusion of the lesion with preservation of the patency and functional validity of the parent vessel (reconstructive operation) or occlusion of the parent vessel at the orifice of the aneurysm (deconstructive operation). The terms "reconstructive" and "deconstructive" operation in the above sense were introduced by Serbinenko (1972, 1974 a, b).

Deconstructive operations are performed when direct attack and the reconstructive balloon catheter procedure proves impossible. It may also be forced upon the surgeon in cases where a reconstructive operation had been planned originally.

Permanent occlusion of the aneurysm is performed by filling the balloon positioned in the aneurysmal cavity with a quickly hardening substance (silicone). The volume of silicone administered depends on the volume and form of the aneurysm. The amount of silicone for adequate occlusion of the aneurysm may vary from 0.1 to 1.0 ml or more. The silicone-filled balloon weakens the force of the sphincter and the balloon becomes immobile due to its cohesion to the aneurysmal walls. The conditions created following filling of the balloon allow free removal of the catheter from the former. As the sphincter may leak fluid, the catheter is removed only after polymerization of the silicone that takes from 3 to 20 minutes. It is not necessary to fill the balloon with silicone to such a degree that the balloon acquires an angiographically visualized form of the aneurysm. It is sufficient to introduce into the balloon as much silicone as necessary to immobilize the balloon (or balloons) in the aneurysm. Immobility of the balloon is achieved when the head end of the silicone-filled balloon touches the aneurysmal wall while the tail, considerably exceeding in size the diameter of the aneurysmal orifice, obliterates completely the neck of the lesion. It has therefore been considered preference in most cases for the silicone-filled balloon to acquire not a spherical but a longitudinally-oval shape (Fig. 1). The length of the catheter depends on the location of the aneurysm and should be sufficient to convey the balloon to the cavity of the aneurysm. The form of the balloon is of prime significance and should vary depending on the need to occlude small or large aneurysms, those with a wide or narrow neck. Experience shows that for "fixation" of the balloon in the aneurysm one usually requires a smaller quantity of silicone than one might expect from the angiographic finding.

IV. Material and Methods

The communication is based on an analysis of 137 intravascular interventions performed by the authors at the Kiev Research Institute of Neurosurgery in 119 patients with saccular aneurysms of the cerebral arteries from November 1974 through December 1980. Postoperative follow-up was from one month to six years.

Summarized data on the number of cases, location of aneurysms, character of the operation and results are presented in the Table. In 67 of the 119 patients the aneurysms were located on the internal carotid artery, namely, cavernous—11, ophthalmic—3, posterior communicating—44, bifurcation—9. In 29 cases the aneurysms were located on the anterior communicating artery, in 22 on the middle cerebral artery: M 1—4, M 2—6, M 3—12 cases. One woman harbored an aneurysm of the posterior inferior cerebellar artery. Multiple saccular aneurysms were revealed in 6 of the 119 patients. The size of the aneurysm varied from 0.3–0.6 to 0.8–3 cm and more. Giant aneurysms (3 cm and more in diameter) were diagnosed in 17 patients. The patients ranged in age from 15 to 65 years and included 77 men and 42 women.

Ninety patients were referred to the hospital after the first an 16 after the second subarachnoid haemorrhage; 10 patients were hospitalized as brain tumor suspects; two patients were suspected of an aneurysm on the basis of neurological symptomatology. One anterior communicating artery aneurysm was

Table 1. *Summary of Saccular Aneurysms of Cerebral Arteries*

Location of aneurysm	Total cases	Aneurysm occluded Patency of parent artery preserved (reconstructive operation)	Occlusion of aneurysm and obliteration of parent artery
Internal carotid artery (67)			
cavernous	11	7	4
ophthalmic	3	2	1
posterior communicating			
artery	44	33	5
bifurcation	9	7	
Anterior communicating artery (29)	29	26	3
Middle cerebral artery (22)			
M-1	4	4	
M-2	6	5	
M-3	12	9	1
Posterior inferior cerebellar artery (1)	1		1
	119	93	15

* Not included in the results except the 3 fatalities of the 6 failures to occlude PCA aneurysm.

revealed incidentally in a patient at angiography performed for head injury. On admission the condition was satisfactory in 104, moderately severe in 10 and severe in 5 patients.

Total rapid serial cerebral angiography was performed in all patients and usually clear information was obtained on the location of the aneurysm, its form and size. Supplementary valuable findings on the size and location of the aneurysmal neck were gained by cineangiography (S. A. Romodanov *et al.* 1979).

V. Indication for Surgery

The intravascular method by means of the detachable balloon catheter opens new horizons both in the prophylaxis and treatment of hemorrhagic stroke and its sequels due to saccular aneurysms of cerebral arteries and other malformations of brain blood vessels. This method enables successful management in cases where major intracranial operations would have to be performed as well as in instances when direct surgery even using modern microsurgical techniques is difficult or impossible (aneurysms of the intracavernous portion of the carotid

Treated by Intravascular Detachable Balloon Catheter Technique

Failure to occlude aneurysm	Results			
	Good	Fair	Poor	Death
	8			3
	3			
6*	36	1	1	3
2	6	1		
	26	1	1	1
	4			
1	4	1		
2	9		1	
	1			
11	97	4	3	7

artery, giant saccular aneurysms etc. We consider detachable balloon catheter surgery for saccular aneurysms of the cerebral arteries to be the least hazardous of the currently existing operations for this type of lesion. When reconstructive surgery by means of the detachable balloon catheter proves impossible the operation is discontinued and the traditional direct intracranial approach may be considered.

At first we used the detachable balloon catheter only for occlusion of those saccular aneurysms of the cerebral arteries that were unapproachable by direct surgery. Reassured by the favourable results we extended the indications for intravascular operations aimed to occlude most types of saccular aneurysms of the cerebral arteries with preservation of patency of the parent vessel.

At present, endovascular surgery for saccular aneurysms of the cerebral arteries is indicated when one establishes angiographically that the location, size of the aneurysm and its neck are approachable for insertion of the detachable balloon.

Our experience indicates that as a rule none of the anatomical localizations should be considered an absolute contraindication for the intravascular manage-

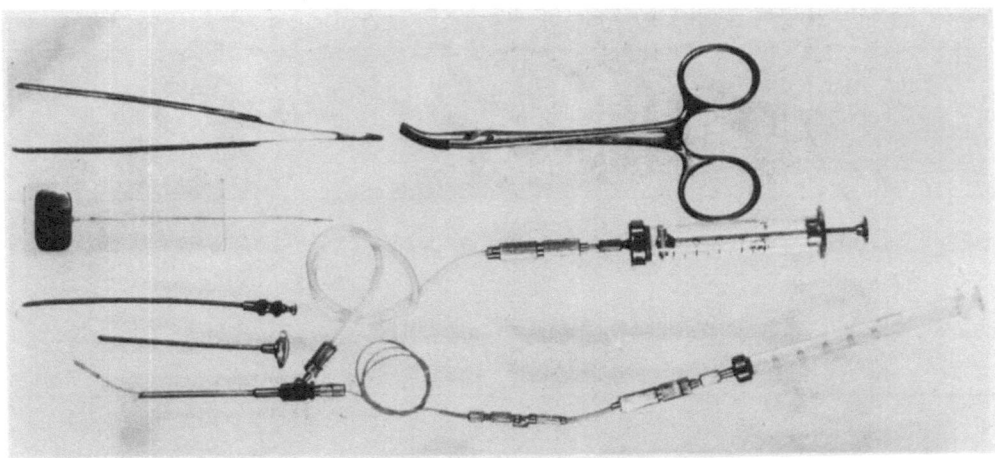

Fig. 3. Instruments for occlusion of saccular aneurysms of cerebral arteries

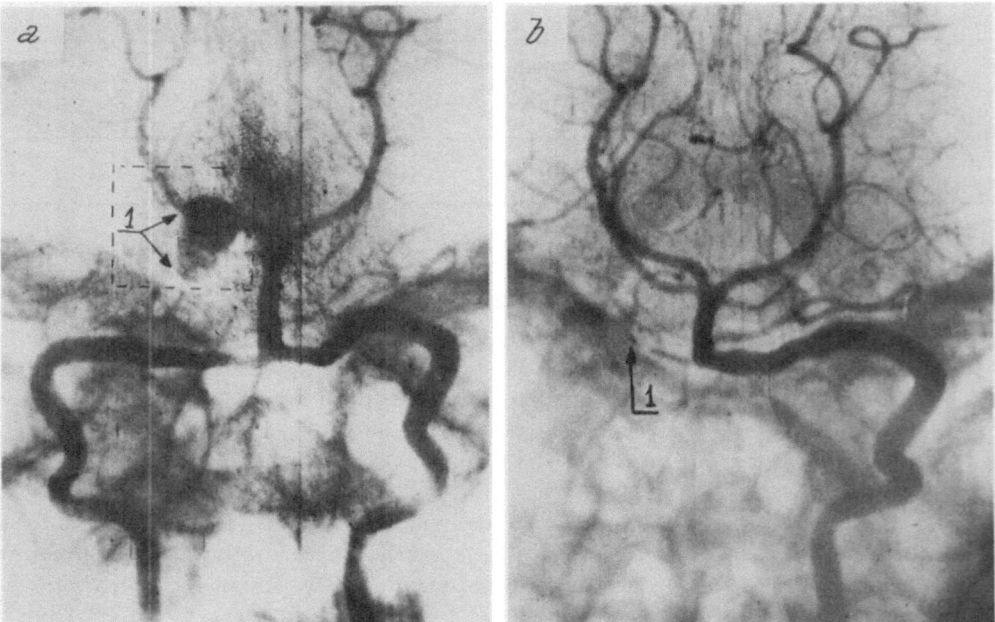

Fig. 4. (a) Posterior inferior cerebellar artery aneurysm (arrows) before the operation in a 16-year-old girl; (b) control angiogram 6 months after the operation showing occlusion of the aneurysm and parent vessels. Arrow shows the balloon mark

ment of saccular aneurysm of the brain arteries. It is, however, difficult at present to draw conclusions about aneurysms of the vertebral artery territory. We have succeeded in occluding only one aneurysm of the posterior inferior cerebellar artery (Fig. 4) without complications.

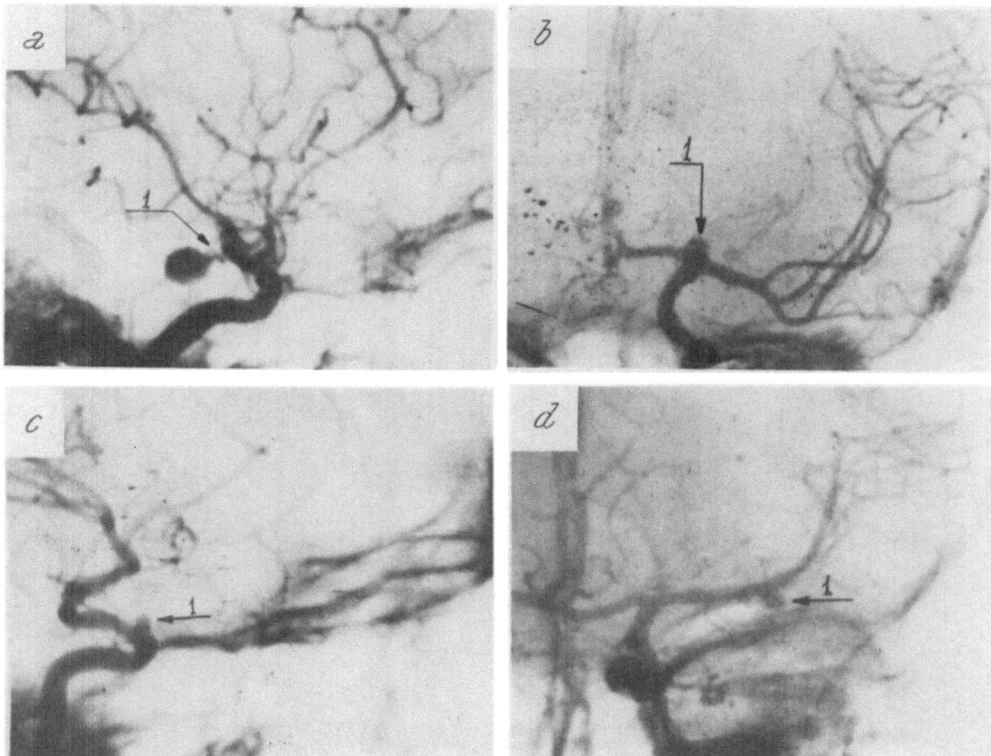

Fig. 5. (a) Supraclinoid aneurysm with a narrow deformed neck; (b) internal carotid artery bifurcation aneurysm with a very large neck; (c) very small-sized ophthalmic aneurysm; (d) very small-sized and narrow-necked middle cerebral aneurysm

The age limit is also not an absolute contraindication to intravascular surgery. The health status of the patient at the time of surgery is here of prime importance. However, the elderly patients (65 years and over) require particular care and a detailed consideration of all gerontological and geriatric problems.

Intravascular surgery is contraindicated in patients with saccular aneurysms of the cerebral arteries in the presence of intracranial hematomas, in small-sized aneurysms unapproachable for insertion of the balloon, in aneurysms with a narrow deformed neck in small aneurysms with a very wide neck (Fig. 5). The intravascular operation is also not indicated in most patients during the acute period of intracranial hemorrhage or in patients showing marked spasm of the cerebral arteries.

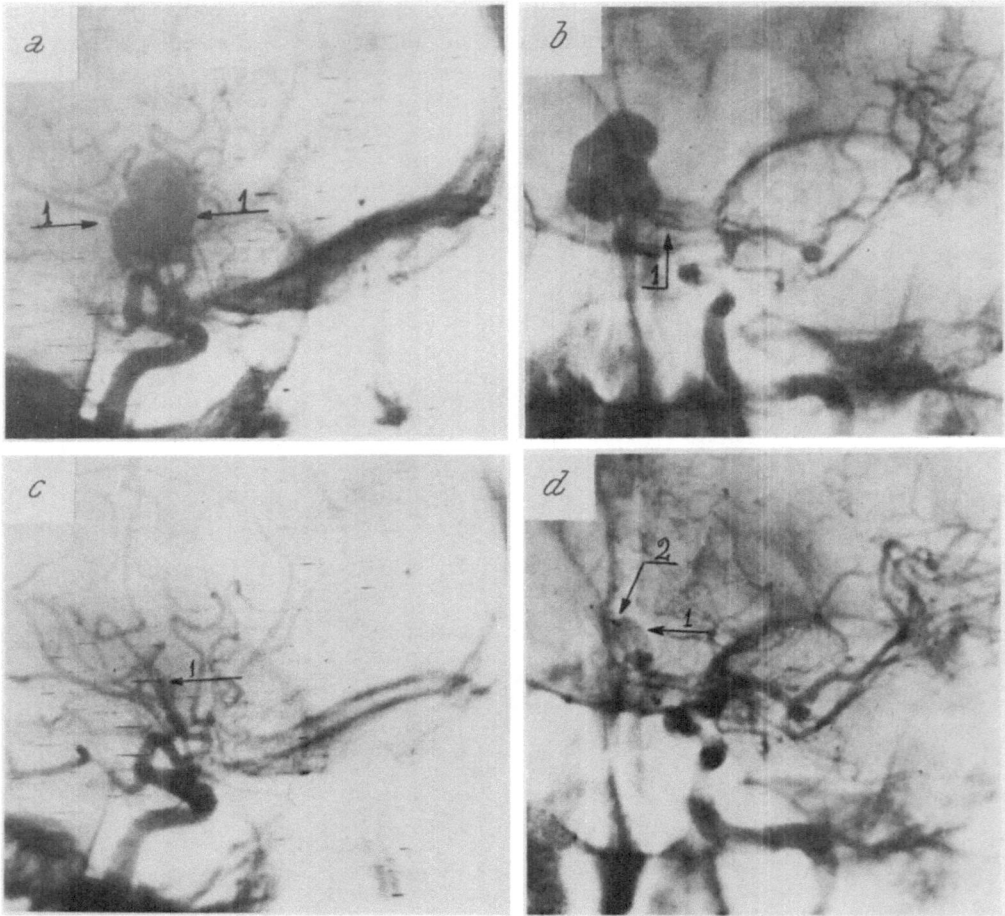

Fig. 6. (a), (b) Large anterior communicating artery aneurysm (arrows) in a 30-year-old
female after the second hemorrhage before the operation; (c), (d) control angiography 17
days after reconstructive surgery: (c) *1* balloon mark; (d) *1* balloon; *2* balloon mark

In patients with a history of intracranial bleeding from the aneurysm the
detachable balloon catheter operation was timed not earlier than 2–4 weeks after
the accident.

In 1980 we performed the first successful occlusion of a saccular cerebral
aneurysm during the acute period with preservation of the parent artery. This
female patient with a large aneurysm of the anterior communicating artery was
operated on the fifth day following a second bleeding (Fig. 6); in a second patient
with a saccular aneurysm of the supraclinoid portion of the carotid artery the
operation was performed on the seventh day following the first bleeding. We
suggest that in the future indications for intravascular aneurysm surgery during
the acute period of subarachnoid bleeding will be extended.

VI. Preoperative Care and the Operation

1. Preoperative Care

The preoperative care is based on a detailed clinical and paraclinical examination of the patient with special emphasis on the functional state of the vascular system. Of particular value for adequate preoperative care are angiographic, electro- and echoencephalographic data, evaluation of rCBF, blood biochemistry, coagulation studies.

Drugs aimed at improving the microcirculation and rheological properties of the blood are of great value in the preoperative period. The patients receive three days and earlier before surgery indirect anticoagulants, aspirin, spasmolytic agents, barbiturates and tranquillizers when necessary. Patients harboring aneurysms accompanied by pituitary-diencephalic disturbances are given corresponding hormones 3-5 days prior to surgery. At present, indirect anticoagulants are administered only 1-2 days before the operation, because longer use may result in some cases in mild but poorly controllable bleeding from the soft tissues of the artery puncture site. Immediately before the operation and during surgery hemodilution is carried out by means of dextrans (rheopolyglukin). The premedication has included promedol, dimedrol, atropine, papaverine, sodium oxybutyrate. All this creates more favourable conditions for the intravascular balloon catheter intervention.

2. The Operation

The operation is begun immediately after hemodilution and procaine block of the upper sympathetic ganglion on the side of the aneurysm. The carotid artery is punctured by a special needle (Fig. 3) with an external diameter of 2-2.2 mm (lumen 1.6-1.8-2.0 mm). These needles are convenient and safe. Their lumen is sufficient for simultaneous easy introduction of 2-4 balloon catheters and for their safe subsequent removal from the circulation. To avoid injury of the endothelium the needle is introduced into the lumen of the common or internal carotid artery by means of a plastic introducer. The balloon catheters are introduced into the needle and guided under continuous monitoring to the site of the aneurysm. One or even two loops of the artery in the neck are not an unsurmountable obstacle for advancing the balloon catheters but in some cases the balloon catheters may have to be filled with a radiopaque substance to increase the pulling force of the balloon. The operation is postponed till the next trial when one fails to puncture the artery adequately.

The intravascular intervention lasts routinely 40-120 minutes. Local anesthesia is usually sufficient for the operation and analgesic and sedative agents are administered additionally during surgery. The operation is, therefore, usually not performed under general anesthesia. Verbal contact with the patient is very important to determine during the stage of temporary occlusion the functional significance of the aneurysm-bearing artery.

After puncturing the carotid artery slow intravenous administration of saline heparin solutions are begun (total dose 15,000-25,000 units). About 5,000-7,000 units of heparin may be administered directly into the punctured carotid artery. In combination with dextran this proves effective in the prophylaxis of the formation of clots in the blood vessels, balloon catheter. needle. After the operation a heparin antidote (protamine sulfate) is given.

During surgery one controls graphically and visually the arterial pressure, pulse, respiration, ECG and EEG, values the neurological status. The systemic arterial pressure is kept at initial levels during surgery.

2.1. Introduction of Balloon Catheters into the Aneurysm

At least three conditions must exist for introducing the balloon catheter into the aneurysmal cavity: a) the diameter of the aneurysm should measure not less than 0.5 cm, the diameter of the neck should not exceed that of the balloon; b) availability of a flexible, elastic balloon catheter with a mobile balloon and tip of the catheter to which the balloon is fastened. The balloon has to be soft, with a smooth oval surface of the head part and preferably with a "heavy" tip. This increases the mobility, flexibility and facilitates movement of balloon not in the blood flow center but closer to the wall of the artery; c) the changed blood stream patterns at the aneurysmal orifice (turbulence) are a condition favouring insertion of the balloon into the aneurysm. This condition may be. if necessary, artificially promoted by special manoeuvering with the supplementary balloon catheters in the region of the aneurysmal orifice. The presence of turbulence and changes of the blood flow linearity at the aneurysmal orifice may be evaluated fluoroscopically and cineangiographically. particularly. in the case of large aneurysms.

Immediately before occlusion of the aneurysm two balloon catheters are introduced into the carotid artery: a detachable and non-detachable. The detachable balloon is introduced into the aneurysm and filled with a small quantity of radiopaque substance and silicone so that the balloon cannot escape through the neck of the aneurysm at detachment of the catheter. The size of the neck is easily determined by means of the non-detachable balloon catheter which is filled with radiopaque substance so as to close the neck of the aneurysm. Ten minutes later the catheter is detached from the balloon. In 10 cases the movements of the detached balloon in the aneurysmal cavity were circular. synchronous with the pulse. The movements of the balloon became irregular following rapid periodic digital compression of the carotid artery. Cessation of balloon movement in the aneurysm was noted after complete temporary occlusion of the carotid artery by a non-detachable balloon. A study carried out by S. A. Romodanov et al. (1979) confirmed the presence of turbulent blood flow in the aneurysm and changes of blood flow linearity at its level. Cessation of movements of the balloon in the aneurysmal cavity confirms arrest of blood flow in it. Chaotic, irregular movements of the balloon in the aneurysmal cavity with a maintained blood flow in the carotid artery (3 cases) may indicate filling defects in the aneurysm, e.g. presence of blood clots. This information is of value for intravascular surgery planning. In most cases the balloon catheter made individually for each patient has been introduced into the aneurysmal cavity without any auxiliary manipulations. Adequately designed balloon catheters

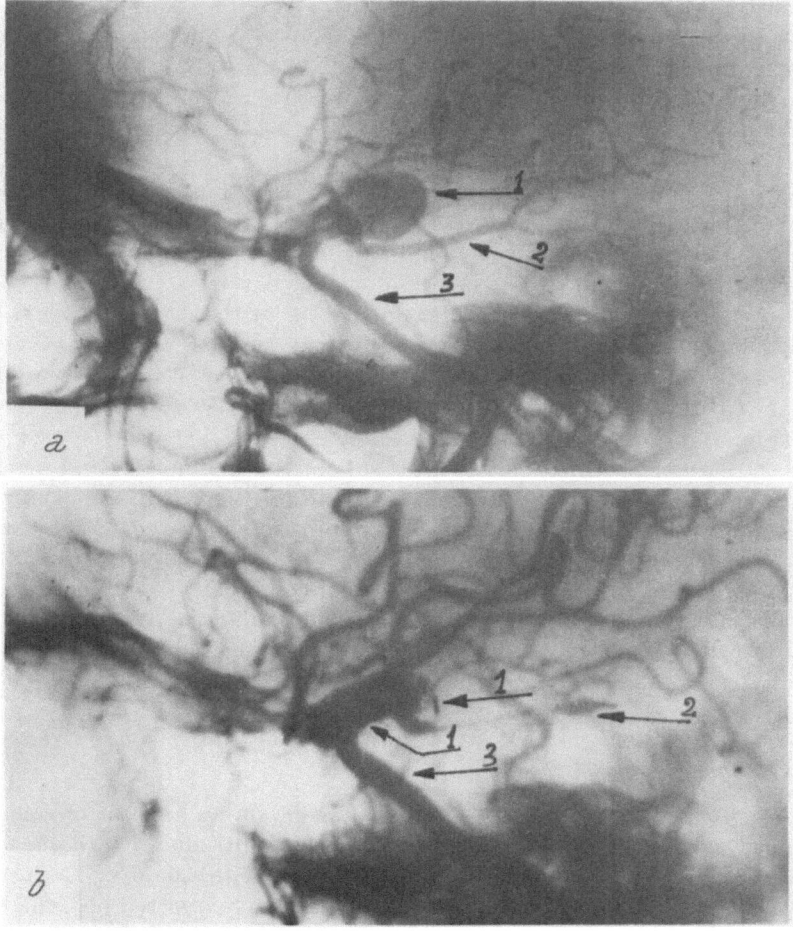

Fig. 7. Posterior communicating artery aneurysm in a 42-year-old male. *1* aneurysm; *2* posterior cerebral artery; *3* internal carotid artery; (b) temporary occlusion of posterior cerebral artery (*2*) to facilitate insertion of balloon catheter into the aneurysm (*1*); *3* internal carotid artery

have been directed into the aneurysm by the blood stream with the help of manoeuvering of the balloon catheters (in 81 of the 119 patients). In the remaining 38 cases we tried to direct the balloon into the aneurysm by various non-standard techniques using one detachable and one or two non-detachable balloon catheters. The detachable catheter is placed at the aneurysmal orifice or several millimeters below it, one non-detachable balloon catheter is placed above the aneurysmal orifice, the second somewhat below the detachable catheter. The plunger of the syringe connected with the detachable balloon catheter is pushed by light movements to facilitate introduction of the balloon into the aneurysm. We could do this in 20 of the above 38 cases. These manipulations had to be frequently performed in aneurysms of the posterior communicating artery region. In cases when the posterior cerebral artery originated from the carotid artery. it was rather difficult to insert the balloon catheter into the aneurysm due to high blood flow in the posterior cerebral artery. To introduce the balloon catheter into the aneurysm in these cases we had to occlude temporarily the posterior cerebral artery in 6 cases (Fig. 7).

For introduction of the balloon catheter into an aneurysm of the ophthalmic artery region or into an aneurysm on the ophthalmic artery proper it was sufficient to occlude temporarily completely or partially the supraclinoid region of the carotid artery above the orifice of the aneurysm.

Of 67 patients harboring saccular aneurysms of the internal carotid artery the balloon catheter was not inserted into the aneurysm in six cases: in three cases due to a narrow neck. in one case because of a deformed neck and in two cases the entire balloon could not be placed in a small aneurysm with a very wide neck (Fig. 5).

Of 22 patients with saccular aneurysms of the middle cerebral artery the balloon was not introduced into the aneurysm in three cases: one small wide-necked aneurysm and two with necks unapproachable even for our smallest balloon catheters.

Usually saccular aneurysms of the anterior communicating artery permitted easy introduction of the balloon (Fig. 8). The balloon was successfully introduced into the aneurysm of all 29 patients with aneurysms of this location.

2.2. Temporary and Permanent Occlusion of Aneurysms by Means of the Detachable Balloon Catheter

After insertion of the balloon into the aneurysm an amount of radiopaque substance necessary to occlude the aneurysm is introduced into the balloon catheter. The substance is then withdrawn and its quantity is accurately measured. Then a similar amount of silicone is slowly injected into the balloon catheter. The entire course of occlusion of the aneurysm is carefully observed fluoroscopically. After polymerization of the injected silicone the catheter is detached and control angiography is performed.

In saccular aneurysms of small and medium size with a neck adequate for the technique but not very large we usually introduce at first into the aneurysm a non-detachable balloon catheter similar in form and size to a corresponding twin detachable balloon catheter. By means of the non-detachable balloon catheter complete temporary occlusion of the aneurysm is performed by a radiopaque substance. the exact amount of silicone required for complete occlusion of the aneurysm and the "behaviour" of the balloon in the aneurysm are determined. The non-detachable balloon is then replaced by the detachable and silicone is administered to achieve complete occlusion of the aneurysm without preliminary administration of radiopaque substance (Fig. 8. 9).

For occlusion of large and giant saccular aneurysms of the cerebral arteries measuring 3 cm and more in diameter (Fig. 10, 11) and usually having wide necks, 2-3 balloon catheters are simultaneously introduced into the aneurysm

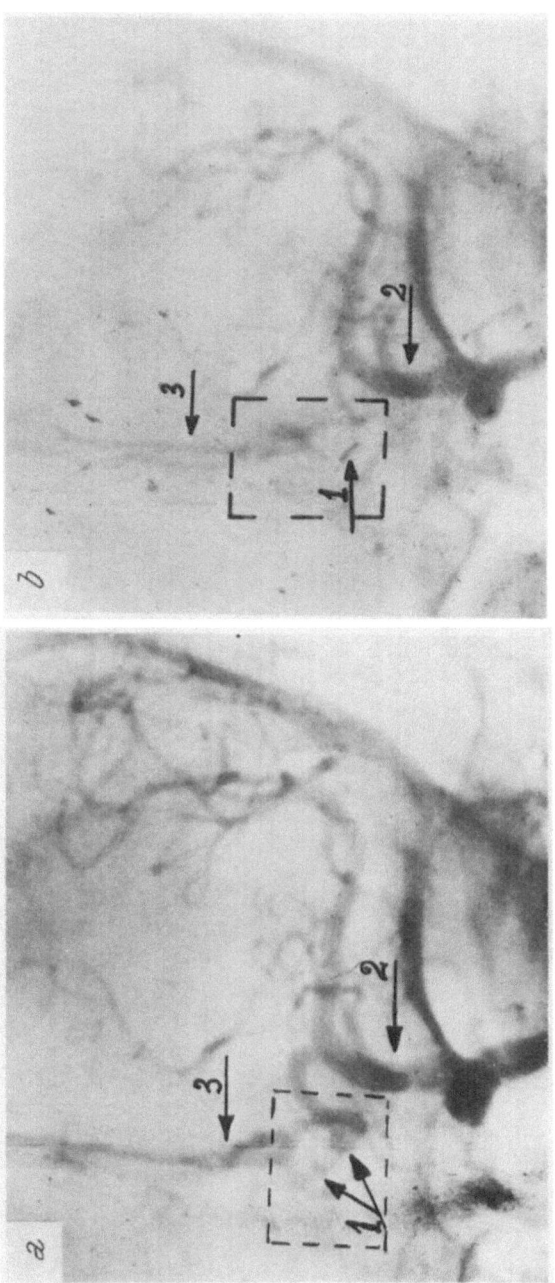

Fig. 8. (a) Small anterior communicating artery aneurysm before the operation in a 23-year-old female (1); 2 internal carotid artery; 3 anterior cerebral artery; (b) control angiography 2 years after operation. Aneurysm occluded by balloon (1); 2 internal carotid artery; 3 anterior cerebral artery

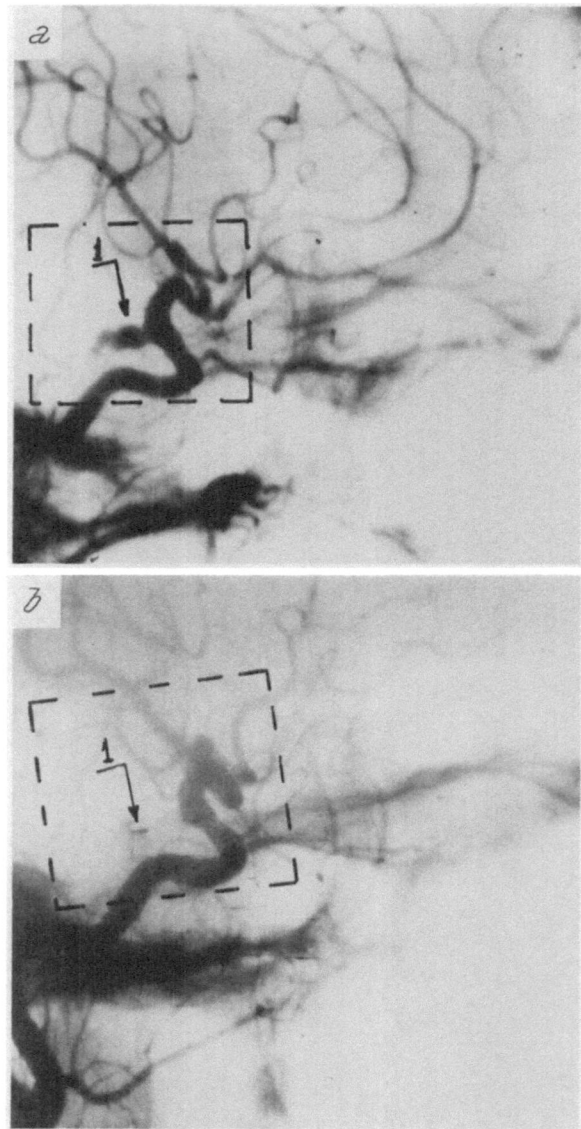

Fig. 9. (a) Supraclinoid aneurysm (*1*) in a 39-year-old female; (b) control angiography immediately after operation; *1* mark of balloon filled only with silicone; *2* internal carotid artery

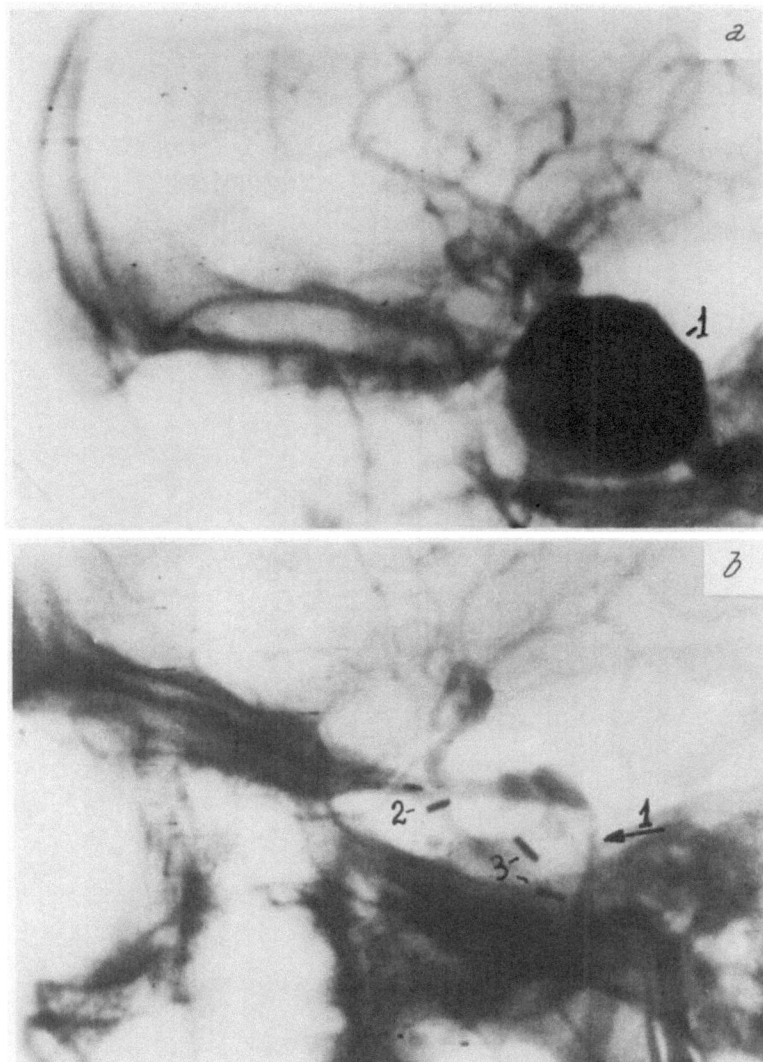

Fig. 10. (a) Giant cavernous carotid aneurysm (*1*) in a 28-year-old female; (b) control angiography 1 year after the operation. Aneurysm occluded by 4 balloons (*2, 3*); *1* internal carotid artery

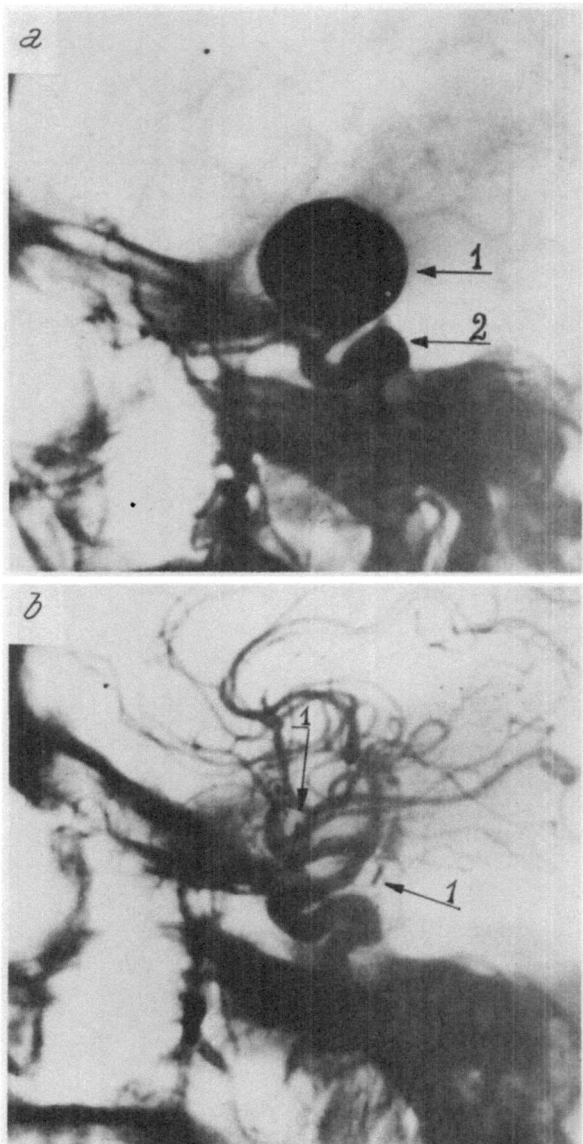

Fig. 11. (a) Large supraclinoid aneurysm (*1*) in 48-year-old female; *2* internal carotid artery; (b) control angiography 1 month after operation. Aneurysm occluded by 2 balloons (*1*)

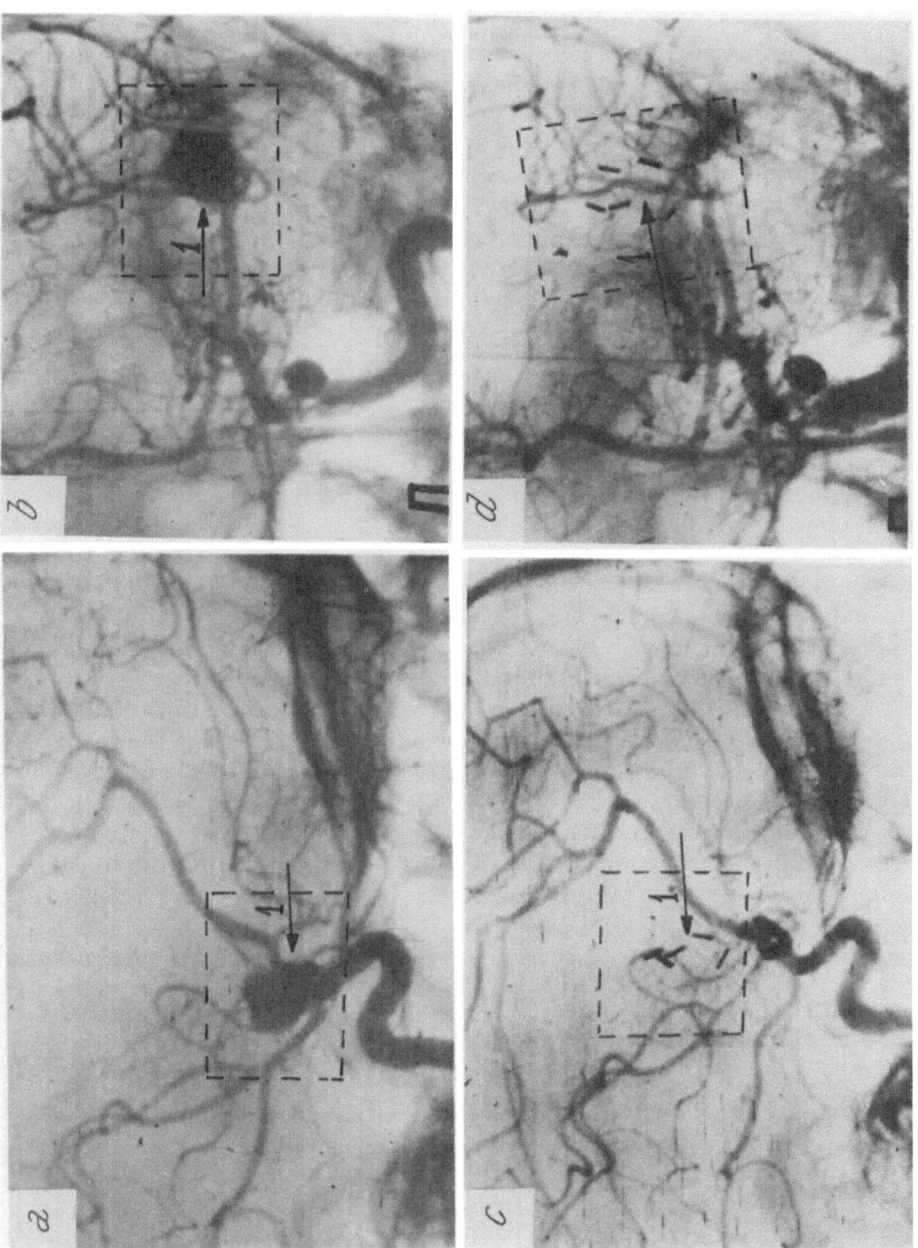

Fig. 12. (a), (b) Middle cerebral artery aneurysm (1) in a 28-year-old male; (c), (d) control angiography 1 year after operation. Aneurysm occluded by 5 ballons (1).

and filled with a radiopaque substance. The balloons are so positioned in the aneurysm as to occlude it and preserve the parent artery. After withdrawal of the radiopaque substance liquid silicone is introduced into the balloon catheters. Consecutive release of the catheters from each balloon is carried out after polymerization of the silicone. When the balloon happens to be smaller than the neck of the aneurysm the balloon may be withdrawn into the lumen of the parent artery during detachment of the catheter and, thus, obliterate the artery at the level of the aneurysmal orifice. To avoid this, exact measurements of the aneurysmal neck should be carried out by the balloon catheter before administration of silicone and a balloon catheter of adequate form and size should be chosen.

When one balloon catheter is not sufficient in the course of temporary obliteration to occlude completely the aneurysm and it proves impossible to introduce other catheters into the aneurysm the first balloon catheter is replaced by several others sufficient to perform a reconstructive operation (Fig. 12).

2.3. Complications

Serious complications caused by the intravascular procedures were mainly observed during the period of development of this new method. These complications include rupture of the aneurysm by the balloon in one case; rupture of the balloon during its filling with silicone resulting in middle cerebral artery thrombosis in one case. These two patients died. In two cases accidental detachment of the balloon from the catheter occurred resulting in thrombosis of some middle cerebral artery branches. These patients developed transient neurological deficit. Unforeseen occlusion of the parent artery occurred in four patients: M-3 branch aneurysm (1), anterior communicating artery aneurysm (1), internal carotid artery aneurysm (2). Only the patient with the M-3 aneurysm showed a permanent neurological deficit. Mild transient neurological disorders developed in the course of intravascular operations for saccular aneurysms of the cerebral arteries in 27 patients. These patients required no special rehabilitation treatment.

Adequate instrumentation, high skill of the neurosurgeon in intravascular techniques, thorough pre- and postoperative care essentially contribute to intravascular surgery without complication using the balloon catheter method. During the last three years we have had no severe complications in our practice.

VII. Results of Intravascular Operations for Saccular Aneurysms of the Cerebral Arteries

Saccular aneurysms have been occluded by means of the detachable balloon catheter in 108 of 119 patients. In 7 patients this could be achieved only after two or three interventions. In 93 patients with occluded aneurysms the reconstructive procedure has been performed: in 49 for aneurysms of the internal carotid artery, in 26 for aneurysms of the anterior communicating artery, in 18 for aneurysms of the middle cerebral artery (Table 1). The deconstructive procedure has been performed in 15 patients: 10, 3, 1, 1 correspondingly for aneurysms of the anterior carotid, anterior communicating, middle cerebral (M-3) and posterior inferior cerebellar artery (Table 1).

The effectiveness of balloon occlusion of the aneurysm was evaluated in all patients angiographically usually after surgery or during the first postoperative days as well as by follow-up repeat angiography 3-6 months and later after surgery (in 87 of the 108 patients). Incomplete recurrence of the aneurysm with radiopaque substance was observed in three cases. One of these patients was reoperated and the aneurysm was completely obliterated by a balloon filled with silicone.

Of the 108 patients in whom occlusion of the aneurysm was performed 4 died (3 after deconstructive and 1 after reconstructive surgery). In three of them the internal carotid artery at the aneurysm level was obliterated by the balloon and the patient died on the third postoperative day due to progressive brain ischemia and edema. The fourth patient with an anterior communicating artery aneurysm died on the ninth postoperative day of pneumonia and development of acute cardio-pulmonary insufficiency.

Of the 11 patients in whom the releasable balloon procedure failed to occlude the aneurysm 3 died, one on the second postoperative day following rupture of a posterior communicating artery aneurysm by the balloon. The second fatality was due to rupture of the balloon during its filling with silicone. The patient with a posterior communicating artery aneurysm died on the ninth postoperative day of middle cerebral artery thrombosis. The third patient died on the 22nd day after surgery following a repeat rupture of the aneurysm, which failed to be occluded by the intravascular procedure.

At discharge from the hospital the condition of the 104 patients operated on by the detachable balloon catheter technique was satisfactory. Of the 8 failures to occlude the aneurysms by intravascular procedures three underwent successful direct intracranial aneurysm surgery using microsurgical techniques and 5 patients refused further surgical treatment. A follow-up study revealed that all 104 patients discharged from the hospital were living and developed no bleeding recurrences. All five patients who refused surgical treatment died of repeated subarachnoid hemorrhage at varying times following discharge from the hospital.

The follow-up results (104 patients) were good (absence of neurological symptoms) in 89 of 92 patients subjected to reconstructive balloon catheter procedures, fair (some neurological deficit; the patients are occupied) in 2 patients and poor in 1 patient who showed neurological deficit before the operation.

In the deconstructive surgery group good results were obtained in 8, fair in 2 and poor in 2 patients.

Conclusion

Data from the literature and our experience with treatment of 119 patients suffering from saccular aneurysms of the cerebral arteries using intravascular procedures by means of detachable balloon catheter indicates that these operations are effective and relatively safe in most cases. We hope that this method of treatment of cerebral arterial aneurysms will find further and wider application in neurosurgical practice.

Acknowledgements

The authors wish to thank K. E. Rudiak for the English translation and J. F. Zemsky for preparing the photographs.

References

Alksne. J. F.. 1968: Magnetically controlled intravascular catheter. Surgery *64*. 339—345.

Brooks. B.. 1930: The treatment of traumatic arteriovenous fistula. South. Med. J. *23*, 100—106.

Debrun. G.. Lacour, P.. Caron, J. P., Hurth, M., Comoy. J., Keravel. J.. 1975: Inflatable and released balloon technique. Experimentation in dog. application in man. Neuroradiology *9*. 267—271.

— — — 1977: Balloon arterial catheter techniques in the treatment of arterial intracranial diseases. In: Advances and Technical Standards in Neurosurgery, Vol. *4* (Krayenbühl. H.. *et al.*. eds.). pp. 131—145. Wien-New York: Springer.

— — — Hurth, M.. Comoy. J., Keravel, J.. 1978: Detachable balloon and calibrated-leak balloon technique in the treatment of cerebral vascular lesions. J. Neurosurg. *49*. 635—649.

Di Tullio, M. V.. Rand, R. W., Frisch. E., 1978: Detachable balloon catheter. Its application in experimental arterio-venous fistulae. J. Neurosurg. *48*, 717—723.

Fogarty. T. J., Granley. J. J., Krause. R. J.. *et al.*. 1963: A method for extraction of arterial emboli and thrombi. Surg. Gynec. Obstet. *116*. 241—244.

Kessler, L. A.. Wholey. M. H.. 1970: Internal carotid occlusion for treatment of intracranial aneurysms. Radiology *95*. 581—583.

Laitinen. L.. Servo. A.. 1978: Embolization of cerebral vessels with inflatable and detachable balloons. J. Neurosurg. *48*, 307—308.

Lazarev. V. A.. Lysachev, A. G.. 1978: First experience of management of cerebral arterial aneurysms by means of the balloon catheter. In: XI Vsesojuznaja konf. molodykh neirokhirurgov. Moscow. p. 156—157 (Russ.).

Luessenhop. A. J., Spence, W. T., 1960: Artificial embolization of the cerebral arteries for the treatment of arterio-venous malformations. JAMA *172*. 1153—1155.

— Velasquez, A. C.. 1964: Observations on the tolerance of intracranial arteries to catheterization. J. Neurosurg. *21*, 85—91.

— 1978: Intravascular approach in neurosurgical management. In: Progress in Neurological Surgery. Vol. *9* (Krayenbühl. H., Maspes, P. E.. Sweet, W. H.. eds.), pp. 267—317. Basel-New York: S. Karger.

Misiuk, N. S.. 1960: A model of an angioblockader. Vopr. nevropatol. i neirokhir. Arkhangelsk, *3*. 83—85 (Russ.).

Romodanov, A. P.. Shcheglov, V. I.. 1979: Endovascular method of excluding from the circulation saccular cerebral arterial aneurysms. Acta neurochir. (Wien) Suppl. *28*. 312—315.

— Zozulia, Yu. A., Shcheglov. V. I., 1975: Intravascular operations with balloon catheter in cerebrovascular disease and brain tumors. In: Mat. konf. posv. 100-letiu rozhd. L. M. Puuseppa. Tartu, 120—123 (Russ.).

— — — 1979: Balloon catheter occlusion of the feeding vessels of arteriovenous malformations of the brain. Zbl. Neurochir. *40*, 21—28.

Romodanov, S. A.. Shcheglov, V. I., Khoziainov, V. V., 1979: Cineangiography in intracranial aneurysms and carotid-cavernous fistulas. In: Klinika i khirurgicheskoie lechenie sosudistoi patologii mozga pri zabolevaniakh nervnoi sistemy. Leningrad. 109—110 (Russ.).

Rothenberg, S. F., Penka, E. J., Conway, L. W.. 1962: Angiotactic Surgery. Preliminary Studies. J. Neurosurg. *19*, 877—883.

Serbinenko, F. A., 1971: Catheterization and occlusion of cerebral major vessels and prospects for the development of vascular neurosurgery. Vopr. neirokhir. *35*. 17—27 (Russ.).

— 1972: Reconstruction of cavernous part of carotid artery in case of carotid-cavernous fistulae. Vopr. neirokhir. *36*, 3—9 (Russ.).

— 1974 a: Occlusion by ballooning of saccular aneurysms of the cerebral arteries. Vopr. neirokhir. *38*, 8—15 (Russ.).

— 1974: Balloon catheterization and occlusion of major cerebral vessels. J. Neurosurg. *41*, 125—145.

Shcheglov, V. I., 1976: Endovascular interventions in neurosurgical pathology. In: Il Sjezd Neirokhirurgov SSSR. Moscow, 558—559 (Russ.).

— 1979: Current possibilities of intravascular operations by means of the detachable balloon catheter in the treatment of some vascular brain diseases. In: Klinika i khirurgicheskoie lechenie sosudistoi patologii mozga pri zabolevaniakh nervnoi sistemy. Leningrad, 19—21 (Russ.).

Taki, W., Handa, H., Yamagata, S., Matsuda, I., Yonekawa, Y., Ikada, Y., Iwata, H., 1979: Balloon embolization of a giant aneurysm using a newly developed catheter. Surg. Neurol. *12*, 363—365.

Wholey, M. H., Kessler, L. A., Boehnke, M., 1972: A percutaneous balloon catheter technique for the treatment of intracranial aneurysms. Acta radiol. *13*, 286—292.

Yodh, S. B., Pierce, N. T., Weggel, R. J., 1968: Montgomery D. B. A new magnetic system for intravascular navigation. Med. Biol. Eng. *6*, 143—147.

Zlotnik, E. I., Sekach, S. P., 1976: Treatment of carotid-cavernous fistulas and internal carotid aneurysms by the Serbinenko method. In: Il Sjezd Neirokhirurgov SSSR. Moscow, 401—402 (Russ.).

Zozulia, Yu. A., Pedachenko, G. A., Shcheglov, V. I., 1977: Intravascular reconstructive operations for some vascular brain lesions. In: 6th Int. Congr. Neurol. Surgery. Sao Paolo, p. 18.

— Shcheglov, V. I., 1976: Experience and employment of intravascular intervention with a balloon catheter in some type of cerebral pathology. Vopr. neirokhir. *1*, 7—12.

Zubkov, Yu. N., 1974: Intravascular surgery for intracranial internal carotid saccular aneurysms. In: Diagnostika i khir. lechenie sosud. zabol. golovnogo mozga. Leningrad, 173—175 (Russ.).

— 1979: Intraarterial interventions for arterial cerebral aneurysms. In: Akt. vopr. neurol., psikhiat. i neirokhir. Riga, 199—200 (Russ.).

Advances in Computerized Tomography

H. Spiess

Neuroradiologisches Institut, Zürich (Switzerland)

With 13 Figures

Contents

Introduction

The complementing of history and neurological examination by supplementary tests has greatly enriched the fields of neurology, neuropediatrics and neurosurgery in particular. The present sophisticated level of neurosurgery would be impracticable without the technological advances made during the past decades. In 1896 the use of X-rays in medicine signalled the beginning of a new era in medical technology with many new possibilities. Besides methods of examination which disturb a patient little or not at all, such as electroencephalography, examination by ultrasonics and isotope scintigraphy, the techniques of air encephalography, introduced by Walter Dandy in 1918, and cerebral angiography, invented by E. Moniz in 1927, represented considerable progress. However, with the more recently developed method of myelography using opaque contrast media, both of these examination methods require contrast media whose effects may be disagreeable and not completely harmless to a patient.

During the past 10 years, the development of computerized tomography (CT) has been extremely rapid. The first publications about CT led one to expect a very powerful method. At present even those bold expectations have been surpassed. CT systems from a model were created by W. H. Oldendorf in 1961. His original design concept could not be implemented at that time because the state of data processing techniques was insufficient to handle the task. The physicist McCormack (1963) and the electrical engineer Hounsfield (1973) were finally able to implement Oldendorf's concept. In 1973 Ambrose published the first clinical results, an important milestone in neuroradiology, and thereby initiated the very rapid development of CT. After the initial phase, where development proceeded in leaps and bounds, the techniques and instruments have become increasingly specialized, as the field of CT has become more established.

In the following report some of the most impressive advances in CT of the past years will be presented. Possibilities for differential diagnosis will be discussed with focus on innovations in examination techniques of minor pathological alterations at the base of the skull and orbit as well as CT findings of spinal and muscular diseases.

1. Examination Techniques

It is beyond the scope of this report to explain the theoretical principles as well as the mathematical—physical concepts of CT. They have been discussed thoroughly in most of the standard works an publications in recent years (*e.g.* Nadjmi *et al.* 1981, Jacobs *et al.* 1980, Radü *et al.* 1980, Oldendorf 1980).

When using CT there are several specific problems regarding its practical application, such as avoiding errors due to the restlessness of the patient, correct positioning and the use of contrast media. For restless patients, *e.g.* small children or mentally confused individuals, a sedative must be administered for a CT examination. If slight sedation is insufficient general anesthesia should be preferred to stronger sedation, particularly with small children, because of the risk of respiratory depression.

For CT examination of the head symmetrical positioning is desirable. Exact positioning is an absolute necessity for examination of the basal area (orbits and bone structures such as the internal auditory meatus) and for minor lateral ventricle asymmetries. This is not always possible in the case of cranial asymmetry as is well known. In order to position as precisely as possible, a preliminary cross-section of the petrous portion of the temporal bone and the orbit area is worthwhile. Slightly slanted positions can then be easily recognized and possibly corrected for the rest of the examination. With most types of apparatus however, optimal corrections are not possible and, of course depend on the experience and skill of the operator.

A variety of methods and head supports have been developed for stereotactic diagnosis and therapeutic operations aided by CT. With these methods it should be possible to make different types of examinations, such as CT, pneumoencephalogram, and angiogram without changing the position of the head (Bergström *et al.* 1976, Mundinger *et al.* 1978, Greitz *et al.* 1980, Lee *et al.* 1980, Shelden *et al.* 1980). In special cases, for direct examinations in vertical planes, the head may be placed in a strongly reclining or inclining position, possibly with simultaneous body support by means of a wedge in the dorsal or abdominal region. Vertical reconstructions (sagittal, coronal and oblique) of the orbit and skull-base can also be more informative. Such examinations are only worthwhile with motionless patients. All software programs require very thin and in part overlapping slices for a correct and accurate reconstruction.

The use of contrast media can considerably improve CT results for the detection of tumours, infectious diseases and blood vessel malformations. As a rule, intravenous contrast media containing iodine are used as bolus or as an infusion at a dose of 0,5 to 1,0 g of iodine per kg of body weight. For the dynamic studies which have recently become possible smaller and repeated bolus quantities with exact timing between injection and subsequent measurement are required. All contrast injections carry the danger of an allergic reaction. No iodine-containing solution should be injected into a patient to iodine allergy. Severe reactions may occur unexpectedly despite all precautions and, therefore, it is advisable to have shock treatment and reanimation equipment close at hand during the examination. Inhalation of Krypton 77 or Xenon is a decidedly more expensive alternative to iodine-containing substances.

Intrathecal introduction of iodine-containing contrast media is possible in combination with CT. In most cases, relatively small doses of contrast media are sufficient. Continuous monitoring of the patient for possible side effects, however, is also necessary. This method lends itself particularly to the examination of the basal cisterns, the area of the cerebello-pontine angle and for functional diagnosis of reabsorption hydrocephalus. Diagnosis of C.S.F. fistulas or of pathological processes in the cervical and thoracic spine is also made easier. If metrizamide is used intrathecally, a dose of 2 ml., isotonic solution is generally sufficient for children and for adults a dose 2–4 times higher is suggested. The injection can be administered shortly before the CT examination if, directly after injection, the patient is placed in an head-down position.

2. Cerebral CT

CT examination of the brain and its neighbouring structures, is at present, undoubtedly the first method of examination for most of the pathologies in this area. The excellent topographic information obtained through CT also makes it essential for neurotraumatology. Limits to the method concern the diagnostic identification of tumours and the experience of the examiner. In our opinion the accuracy of pathological diagnosis has improved only slowly since 1976, in spite of significantly improved imaging systems. The last 2–3 years in particular, have shown no marked improvement in the diagnostic potential. CT diagnosis can, in our opinion, give correct results, at most, in 50% of cases for the orbit (excluding the globe) and 70–80% of the time for the brain (Spiess 1979, Fuchs 1980).

2.1. Differential Diagnosis Concerning Diffuse Hypodense Changes in the Parenchyma

Reduction in X-ray absorption is found, generally, with the diminution of fibrous constituents and destruction of tissue as well as in cases of water or fat deposits.

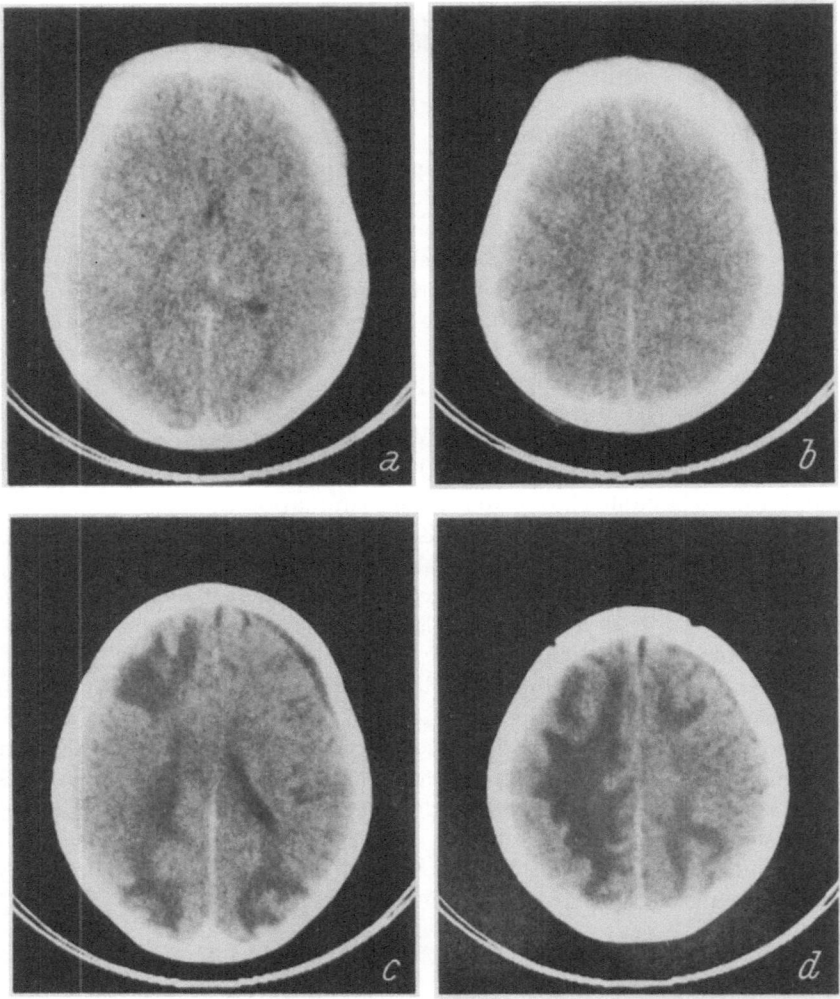

Fig. 1 a–d. a), b) Acute head injury in a 9-year-old girl with moderate brain oedema. c), d) 4 weeks later we see extensive asymmetrical hypodensities in the white matter probably due to hypoperfusion

The absolute density depends largely on the type of CT apparatus being used and on its calibration at anyone time. Absolute values, therefore, cannot be compared. It is better, consequently, to compare only differences in density.

Most types of apparatus measure values between 35 and 45 CT units for the grey matter and between 25 and 35 CT units for the white matter. After addition of contrast media the value is on average 2–5 CT units higher. We measured the average difference between the grey and white matter on the original picture at 6–10 CT units. Values for children were somewhat lower than for older patients. The entire CT diagnosis is based on topography and density values, respectively on the deviation from the normal condition and on the changes after contrast media.

Diffuse hypodense modifications of the parenchyma and their differential diagnosis will now be discussed in greater detail, with the accent on babies and small children.

Probably parallel to the immaturity of the brain, premature births show a predominantly frontal subcortical diminution in density, often in connection with frontal and temporal expansions of the subarachnoid space. This density diminution disappears in the first 3-4 months after birth (Murakami *et al.* 1981).

In the case of full-term births similar density diminutions are found in the white matter, with a certain frontal emphasis in cases of cerebral hypoxia. In cases of serious hypoxia the density is markedly reduced and this change may also reach cortical structures (Flodmark *et al.* 1981).

Through CT we were able to monitor, for a few weeks to a year after birth, 42 cases of subcortical density diminution probably caused by hypoxia. Those cases, where the density on the first examination 1-10 days after hypoxia had diminished by more than 10 CT units (12 cases) never returned to total normality in CT findings. Apart from rare residual density diminution, we saw predominantly expansion of the internal and external CSF spaces. In the cases of density diminution of 5-10 CT units (20 cases), 12 cases (60%) were later found to be normal. Of the 10 cases of slight density diminution up to 5 CT units, only 2 cases (20%) later showed, slightly expanded CSF spaces.

It may be difficult to differentiate the CT appearances of hypoxic encephalo-pathy from those seen in cases of endotoxic encephalopathy (Yong *et al.* 1981); encephalitis; leucodystrophy and traumatic brain oedema, as well as from certain forms of congenital muscular dystrophy (Yoshioka *et al.* 1981). In one of our cases of skull/brain trauma with oedema, probably through a pressure-caused hypoperfusion, a diffuse, predominantly subcortical density diminution appeared within a few weeks (Fig. 1). Similar findings were also described in a diving accident (Nadjmi *et al.* 1981), and we have seen the same after methadone poisoning. In adults, chronic subcortical vascular encephalopathy should be included in differential diagnosis.

For individual cases decisive information concerning severity, type and possible prognosis of the illness is obtainable through CT. For final diagnostic classification, however, the complete history and clinical data are required.

2.2. Orbital Processes

Shortly after CT was introduced it proved to be particularly useful for the examination of the retrobulbar cavity and the periorbital structures. CT diagnosis of the globe proved less successful. Not until the resolution and software programs for reconstruction and high resolution were improved, was some progress achieved. Detection of slight choroidal abnormalities and, in particular, exact location of tumours penetrating the globe and of foreign bodies became possible.

According to our own research (Bigar *et al.* 1981), echography is the preferred method, due to the accuracy of the information obtained for tissue diagnosis in

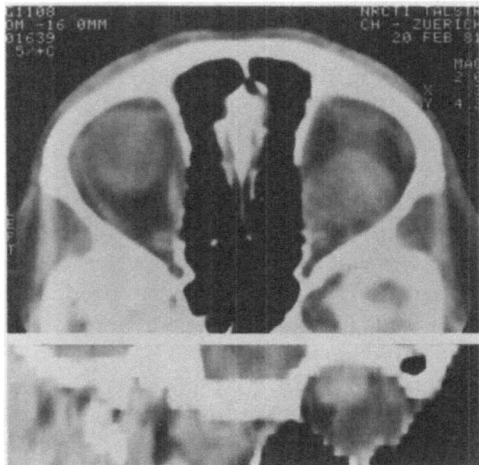

Fig. 2. Malignant lymphoma in the right upper retrobulbar space horizontal slice and
sagittal reconstruction without overlapping slices

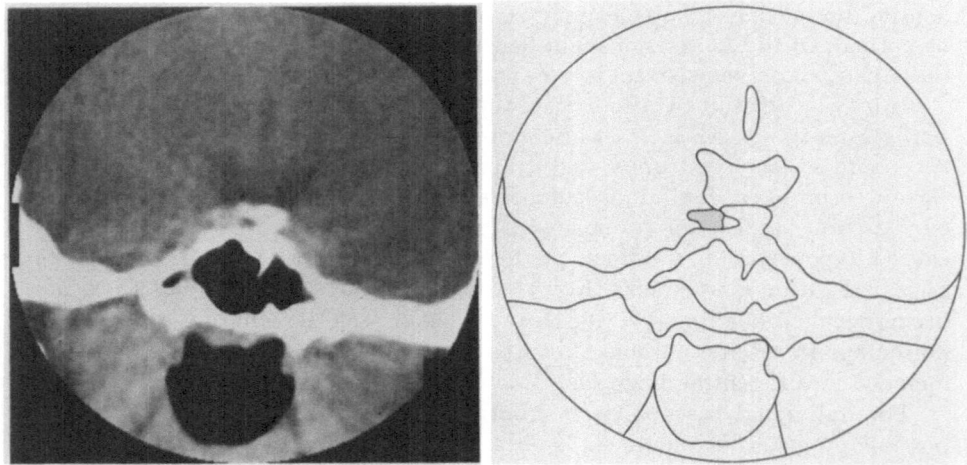

Fig. 3. Intrasellar Prolactinoma, hyperdense, with partial bone destruction

cases of involvement of the anterior third of the orbit. Through CT, additional
information is obtainable if the findings are unclear. In the central third of the
orbit echography and CT are equally precise, whereas towards the rear and in
the periorbital structures the precision of and information from CT is far greater.
The anatomically precise image of the orbit obtained by using thin slices in CT is
amazing (Fig. 2). Traumatic lesions of the limits of the orbit can also be
accurately depicted (Zilkha *et al.* 1981). The application of intravenous contrast
media is rarely needed compared to cases in the interior of the skull.

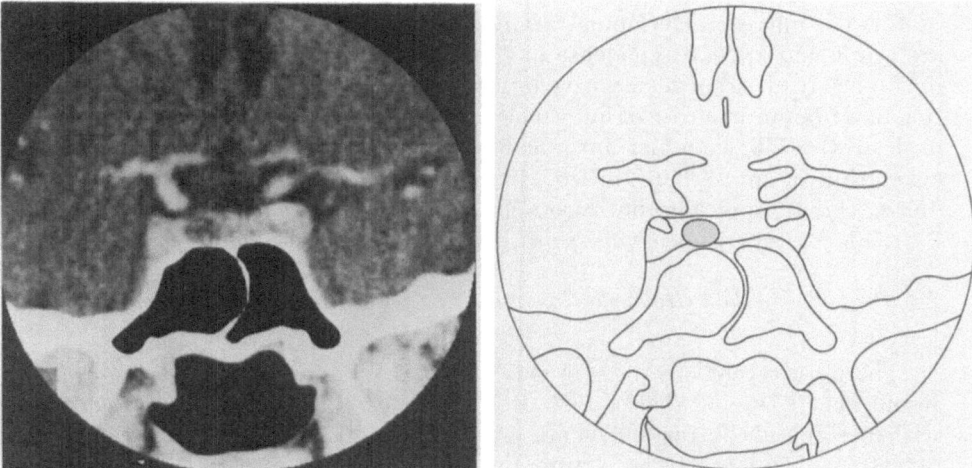

Fig. 4. Purely intrasellar hypodense Prolactinoma (4–5 mm diameter). Acknowledgements: We thank Dr. O. Schubiger, Röntgeninstitut Kantonsspital Aarau for this picture

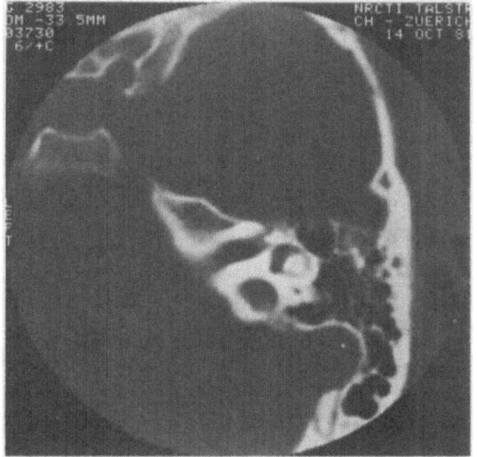

Fig. 5. High resolution picture of the right temporal bone. Note *e.g.* the excellent delineation of the horizontal semicircular canal

2.3. Sellar Processes

Conventional CT can easily detect tumours of the sellar region growing in the para- or suprasellar region. In the case of an intrasellar tumour a convexity in the diaphragm sellae is detectable by CT with intrathecal administration of metrizamide. The so called empty sella is also demonstrable. Reliable detection by CT is not yet possible for micro tumours positioned wholly in the sella and often lacking in bony sellar change. In the absence of calcification, there is a minimum tumour size of 3–5 mm in diameter which is detectable by CT.

Smaller micro-prolactinomas are not detectable. Frequently these tumours are cystic and appear hypodense in CT. Even using an optimal technique one must beware of erroneous positive interpretation in micro-prolactinoma. Detection of a tumour in a case of known elevated serum prolactine values should not mislead the CT examiner into making an over-interpreted diagnosis. The evaluation of intrasellar "micro" findings requires not only much patience during the examination, but also a great deal of experience in interpretation. Particularly important is very thin slicing in the coronal plane (Fig. 3 and 4).

2.4. Processes in the Petrous Portion of the Temporal Bone and the Cerebellopontine Angle Area

The most recent advances in this region are found predominantly in high-resolution CT (Fig. 5, Shaffer 1980, Rettinger et al. 1981) and in its combined use with intrathecal contrast media (air or metrizamide). These procedures allow the detection of inflammatory, traumatic and tumorous processes in the petrous bone itself and, in minor, partly intracanalicular, neurinomas of the acoustic nerve. Should no abnormalities be found during a first, conventional examination, or at most a slightly enlarged meatus acusticus internus, it is worthwhile repeating the examination with intrathecal air or metrizamide injection (Grepe et al. 1978, Hilal 1981).

Thin slicing and high resolution techniques help reduce the otherwise common artefacts in this region.

2.5. Blood-Vessel Malformations

In classical neuroradiology, arteriography with subtraction and angiotomography continues to be the preferred method for the detection of blood-vessel malformations. Undoubtedly, angiography will be necessary prior to any operation. A considerable number of small vessel malformations (saccular aneurysms and angiomas) can be, at present, clearly detected by CT. The additional detection of the size and topography of a haemorrhage as well as accompanying infarcts and subsequent CSF resorption disturbances, represent an additional advantage of CT (Hindmarsh 1977). In acute bleeding however, the fresh blood often veils small vessel malformations, which can be detected by CT only weeks later. The programs at present available for dynamic studies also provide improved diagnostic techniques for vessel malformations and the rate of blood flow through them. The non invasive CT can also be used advantageously for subsequent controls after aneurysm bleeding.

3. Body-CT

3.1. Spinal Processes

Contrary to the view still partly held (Hübener 1981), CT lends itself extremely well to the detection of many spinal processes. Together with high-resolution CT, (Peyster 1981) additional intravenous or intrathecal administration of contrast media may, in part, be required. Questions stated as precisely as possible are a prerequisite to CT examination. If no accurate clinical information as to the height of the lesion is available, classical myelographic methods are still preferable.

In CT of the cervical and thoracic segments of the spinal column, artefacts partly disturb the picture. These are caused primarily by the shoulders and air in the lungs. The artefacts in the cervico-thoracic area are particularly awkward. In the upper cervical region, respectively, in the cranio-cervical area, artefacts caused by tooth fillings must occasionally be by-passed by a special inclination of the gantry. CT provides, for all segments of the spine, a thorough representa-

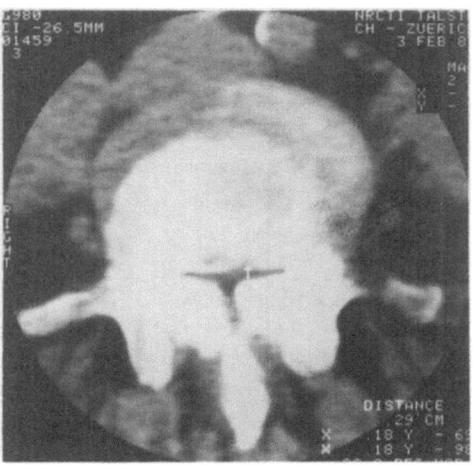

Fig. 6. Extreme narrowing of the lumbar spinal canal

tion of the osseous structures, with possible constrictions and malformations of the spinal canal (Fig. 6).

With enlargement of the CT picture, to correspond to the natural size, the diameters of the spinal canal in all directions can be measured simply with a ruler. Meningomyeloceles and diastematomyelias, and enlargements of the spinal canal caused by tumours (Rusztyn et al. 1981), are also clearly recognized.

The above mentioned artefacts play a minor role in the portrayal of osseous structures. This is not so when assessing the contents of the spinal canal. In our experience, plain examinations of the cervico-thoracic regions alone are often insufficient. Intravenous or intrathecal application of contrast media is often helpful (Fig. 7) as, for example, to demonstrate a syringomyelia (Chuang et al. 1981).

Metrizamide studies of the lumbar region are seldom required today (Vaisman et al. 1981, Gado 1981). Even without contrast media, disc hernias are better recognized than with the conventional myelogram (Fig. 8). This does not apply only to extreme lateral hernias which cannot be detected through myelography (Fig. 9).

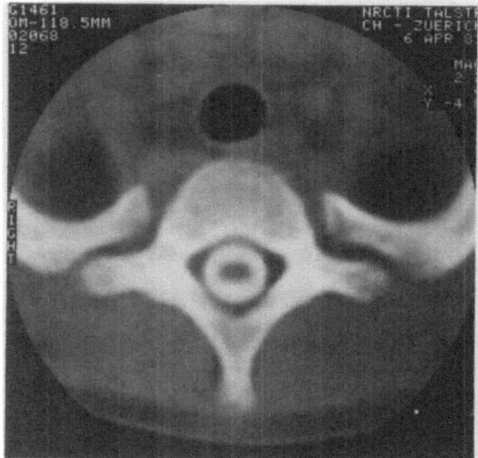

Fig. 7. Metrizamide-CT of the upper thoracic spine. Normal situation

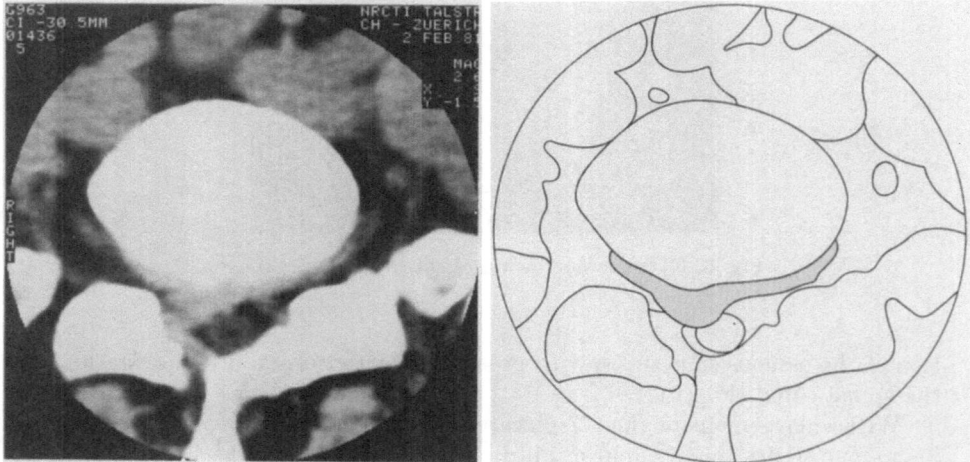

Fig. 8. Recurrent disc herniation L 4/5, mediolateral right

For the examination, slanting of the gantry in the plane of the disc to be examined is required. In the lumbo-sacral position this may not always be possible, because of hyperlordosis. The segments examined should be projected onto the scout view for the neurosurgeon. Clinical experience requires 2-3 disc heights to be examined, depending on the symptomatology. Negative findings in a disc region require the additional examination of segments bordering on the vertebrae examined. As a result, tumours or disc herniae which have luxated upwards or downwards can be detected (Fig. 10). The more thorough the investigation performed by the clinician, the better will be the results.

In operated cases it may be difficult to decide whether a recurrent hernia or

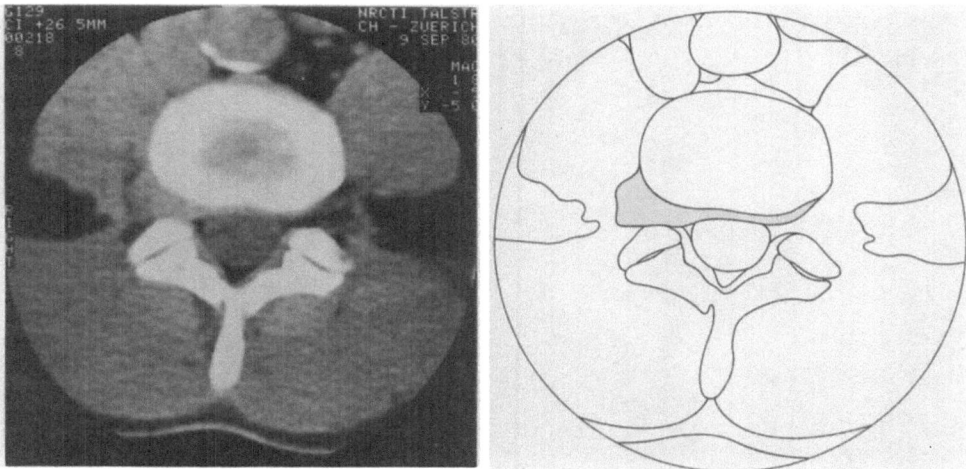

Fig. 9. Extremely lateral disc herniation L 4/5 right

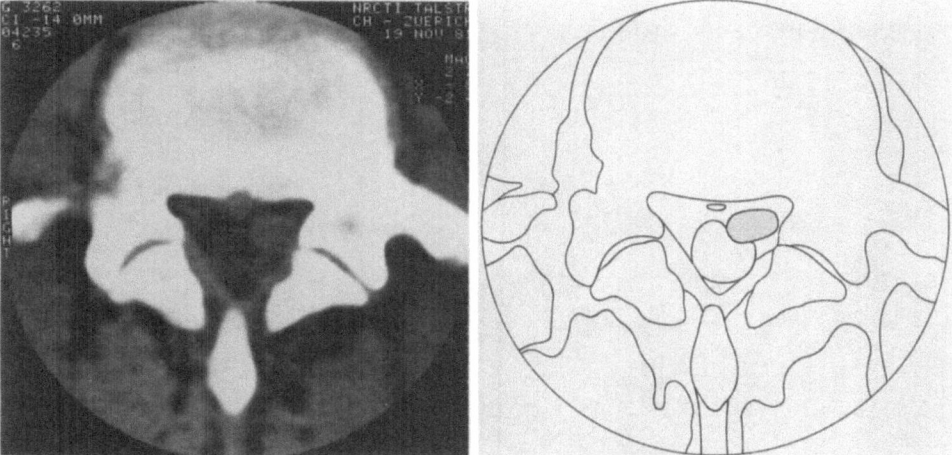

Fig. 10. Downward luxation of disc material left L 4/5 with compression of the dural sack

scar tissue is present. An accurate distinction between the two is not always possible. Scar tissue is likely if the enlarged dural sac in the laminectomy region is surrounded by homogenous, slightly hyperdense tissue and is not, or only slightly, deformed and possibly even distorted towards the side of the operation. A disc relapse with more or less extended scar tissue is likely if limited compression and shifting of the dural sac by non-homogenous tissue is present (Fig. 11 and 12). In more than 50 operated cases we have tried to achieve further differentiation through intravenous contrast media—as suggested by Schubiger *et al.* 1981. Generally scar tissue shows a density increase of 20–50 CT units after the use of a contrast medium. In some cases this may produce additional

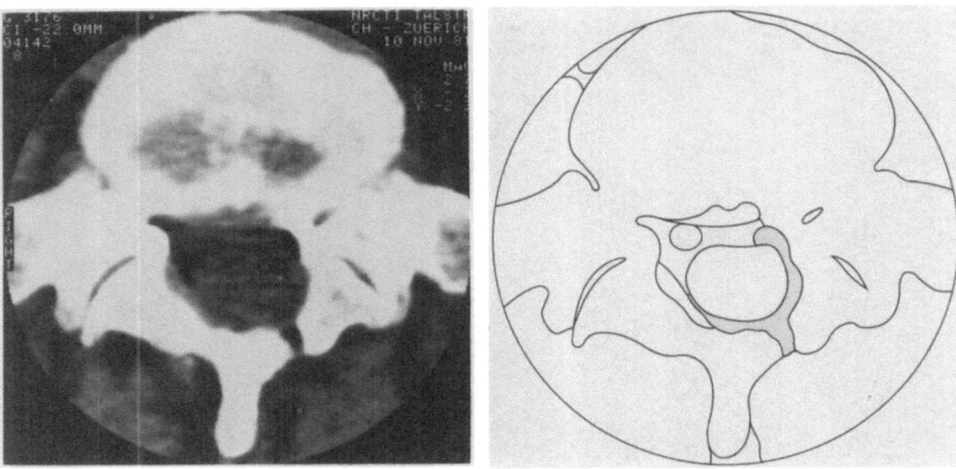

Fig. 11. Hypertrophic scar tissue after operation of disc herniation L5/S1 left. No recurrent herniation. The dural sack is pulled to the left

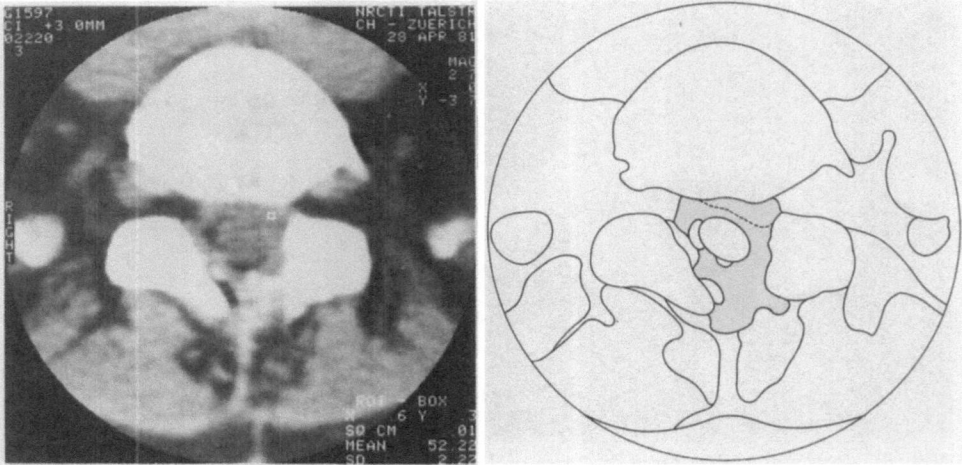

Fig. 12. Hypertrophic postoperative scar tissue plus recurrent herniation with partial compression of the dural sack

diagnostic indication, as usually enhancement is not expected from disc material. This, however, may not differentiate scar tissue combined with a recurrent disc or exclude a new disc prolapse. Comparable density measurements may be inaccurate because of the slightest displacement of the patient or the plane of analysis.

In the diagnosis of disc hernia we should bear in mind the possibility of double hernias. Detection of a lumbosacral hernia should not prevent additional examination of at least disc L4/5. Our experience with CT suggests a less frequent occurrence of authentic double herniae than had been assumed so far on the basis of myelographic examinations. We found authentic double hernias (*i.e.* not merely disc protrusions) in only 4–5% of our cases.

3.2. Neurogenic and Myopathic Muscle Atrophy

In 1979 a standard model for the examination of muscle in healthy persons as well as standard values for the measurement of individual muscles in different age groups, and in part, for the two sexes, had already been suggested and presented (Bulcke *et al.* 1979, 1981).

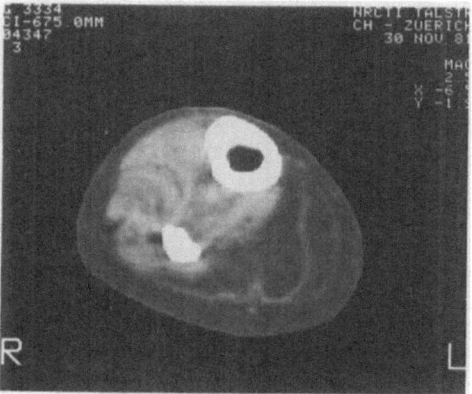

Fig. 13. Scapuloperoneal muscular dystrophy. Cross section through the right lower leg. Extensive fatty degeneration of the gastrocnemius muscle. Previously negative biopsy in this place

The comparison of absolute values is questionable because of the reasons previously stated pertaining to the technical characteristics of the instruments. The difference in density of individual muscles will probably be more distinct between clinically affected and healthy muscle. Recently the CT findings in 3 cases of muscular dystrophy were presented (Bulcke *et al.* 1981). We ourselves compared various cases of neurogenic and myopathic atrophy of muscle particularly with healthy muscle. The cases examined were affected with neurogenic muscle atrophy, *i.e.* affection of the anterior horn (status after poliomyelitis, ALS), radicular and polyradicular atrophy and polyneuropathy (diabetic, alcoholic). Also present were primary muscle affections, individual cases of ocular muscular dystrophy, scapulo-peroneal muscular dystrophy, dystrophia myotonica of Steinert, lipid storage myopathy and one case of paraneoplastic polymyositis.

As the degree of muscular atrophy increases, diffuse or maculated hypodensities which correspond to the fatty degeneration of muscle tissue are found both in the neurogenic and the myopathic group. CT can depict a representative cross-section of muscle atrophy quickly, both for a control examination or as a guide for the appropriate biopsy area in advanced cases of pseudohypertrophy (O'Doherty *et al.* 1977). By using CT, so-called negative biopsies, from which only fat tissue is obtained, can certainly be avoided (Fig. 13). In the case of a lipid storage myopathy, comparatively lower CT-values than in other myopathies were found for clinically apparently intact muscle.

References

Ambrose, J., 1973: Computerized transverse axial scanning (tomography). Part 2. Clinical application. Brit. J. Radiol. *46*, 1023—1047.

Bergström, M., Greitz T., 1976: Stereotaxic computed tomography. Amer. J. Roentgenol. *127*, 143—155; 167—170.

Bigar, F., Spiess, H., 1981: Kombinierte Anwendung der CT und Echographie bei Erkrankungen des Auges und der Orbita. Deutscher Röntgen-Kongreß München.

Bulcke, J. A., Termote, J.-L., Palmers, Y., Crolla, D., 1979: Computed tomography of the human skeletal muscular system. Neuroradiology *17*, 127—136.

— Crolla, D., Termote, J.-L., Baert, A., Palmers, Y., von den Bergh, R., 1981: Computed tomography of muscle. Muscle and Nerve *4*, 67—72.

Chuang, S., Rusztyn, A., Fitz, Ch. R., Harwood-Nash, D., 1980: Metrizamide Myelography in Syringohydromyelia. CT/T Clinical Symposium *3*, Nr. 9.

Cormack, A. M., 1963: Representation of a function by its line integrals, with some radiological applications. J. Appl. Phys. *34*, 2722—2727.

Dandy, W. E., 1919: Roentgenography of the brain after the injection of air into the spinal canal. Ann. Surg. *70*, 397—403.

Flodmark, O., Scotti, G., Harwood-Nash, D. C., 1981: Clinical significance of ventriculomegaly in children who suffered perinatal asphyxia with or without intracranial hemorrhage: An 18 month follow-up study. J. Comput. Assist. Tomogr. *5* (5), 663—673.

Fuchs, M. A., 1980: Hirntumoren in der Computertomographie, Dissertation Zürich 1980.

Gado, M. H., 1981: CT Evaluation of lumbar disc disease: The relative merits of plain and metrizamide studies. International Symposium and Course on Computed Tomography, New Orleans.

Greitz, T., Bergström, M., Boethius, J., Meyerson, B., Collins, V. P., 1980: Stereotactic Biopsy of Cerebral Lesion. CT/T Clinical Symposium, *3*, Nr. 7.

Grepe, A., Greitz, T., Norén, G., 1978: Computer cisternography of extracerebral tumors using lumbar injection of water soluble contrast medium. Acta radiol. (Diagn.) Suppl. *346*, 51—62.

Hilal, S. K., 1981: Study of cerebellopontine angle with metrizamide and high resolution CT. International Symposium and Course on Computed Tomography, New Orleans.

Hindmarsh, T., Greitz, T., 1977: Hydrocephalus, atrophy and their differential diagnosis—(CSF dynamics investigated by computer cisternography). In: Computerized Axial Tomography in Clinical Practice (du Boulay, G. H., Moseley, I. F., eds.), pp. 205—212. Berlin-Heidelberg-New York: Springer.

Hübener, K. H., 1981: Computertomographie des Körperstammes, Röntgen wie? wann? Band VI (Frommhold, W., Hrsg.). Stuttgart-New York: Thieme.

Hounsfield, G. N., 1973: Computerized transverse axial scanning (tomography). Part 1. Description of system. Brit. J. Radiol. *46*, 1016—1022.

Jacobs, L., Weisberg, A., Kinkel, W. R., 1980: Computerized Tomography of the Orbit and Sella Turcica. New York: Raven Press.

Lee, S. H., Villafana, T., Lapayowkeri, M. S., 1980: CT: Intracranial localisation with a new marker system. Neuroradiology *16*, 570—571.

Moniz, E., 1927: L'encéphalographie arterielle. Son importance dans la localisation des tumeurs cérébrales. Rev. Neurol. (Paris) 72—90.

Mundinger, F., Birg, W., Ostertag, C. B., 1978: Treatment of small cerebral gliomas with CT-aided stereotaxic Curie therapy. Neuroradiology 16, 564—567.

Murakami, R., Nakamura, H., Mizojiri, T., Aida, M., Matsuo, T., 1981: A study of brain development in low-birth-weight infants by computerized tomography. Neuropediatrics 12, 132—142.

Nadjmi, M., Piepgras U., Vogelsang, H., 1981: Kranielle Computertomographie. Stuttgart-New York: Thieme.

O'Doherty, D. S., Schellinger, D., Raptopoulos, V., 1977: Computed tomographic patterns of pseudohypertrophic muscular dystrophy: Preliminary results. J. Comput. Assist. Tomogr. 1, 482—486.

Oldendorf, W. H., 1961: Isolated flying-spot detection of radiodensity discontinuities; displaying in the internal structural pattern of a complexe object. IEEE-Trans. Biomed. Electron 8, 68—72.

— 1980: The Quest for an Image of Brain. New York: Raven Press.

Peyster, R. G., 1981: High resolution CT scanning of the spine. International Symposium and Course on Computed Tomography, New Orleans.

Rettinger, G., Kalender, W., Hentsche, F., 1981: Hochauflösungs-Computertomographie des Felsenbeines. Computertomographie 1, 109—116.

Radü, E. W., Kendall, B. E., Moseley, I. F., 1980: Computertomographie des Kopfes. New York: Thieme.

Rusztyn, A., Chuang, S., Fitz, Ch. R., Harwood-Nash, D., 1981: Meningomyelocele with Diastematomyelia. CT/T Clinical Symposium 3, Nr. 13.

Schubiger, O., Valavanis, A., Dabir, K., Imhof, H. G., 1981: CT-Differentiation between recurrent disc herniation and postoperative scan-formation: The value of contrast enhancement. X. Congress of the European Society of Neuroradiology, Milan.

Shaffer, K., 1980: Cholesteatoma. CT/T Clinical Symposium 3, Nr. 13.

Shelden, C. H., McCann, G. D., Jacques, S., Lutes, H., Frazier, R., Katz, R., Kubci, R., 1980: Development of Computerized Microstereotactic Method for the Localisation and Removal of Minute CNS Lesions under direct 3-D Vision, J. Neursurg. 52, 21—27.

Spiess, H., 1979: CT-Ergebnisse bei Affektionen des Chiasmas und der Sehbahn. Klin. Mbl. Augenheilk. 174, 816—829.

Vaisman, U., 1981: Herniated Disc in the Lumbar Spine. CT/T Clinical Symposium 4, Nr. 7.

Yong, R. S. K., Towfighi, J., Yagel, S. K., Vanucci, R. C., 1981: Neonatal endotoxin Encephalopathie: Physiologic, Metabolic and Neuropathologic responses. American Academy of Neurology, 33rd annual meeting.

Yoshioka, M., Okuno, R., Ito, M., Konishi, Y., Itagaki, Y., Sakamoto, Y., 1981: Congenital muscular dystrophy (Fukuma Type). Repeated CT studies in 19 children. Comp. Tomography 5, 81—88.

Zilkha, A., 1981: Computed tomography in trauma to the orbital walls. International Symposium and Course on Computed Tomography, New Orleans.

B. Technical Standards

Surgical Approaches to the Tentorial Hiatus

L. Symon

Gough-Cooper Department of Neurological Surgery, Institute of Neurology (London University) and the National Hospital, London (Great Britain)

With 26 Figures

Contents

Introduction

Access to the tentorial hiatus presents the neurological Surgeon with more than usual difficulty. In addition to the depth of the exposure, and the necessity for considerable retraction of overlying brain, lesions lying in the region of the hiatus tend to involve vital areas of the brain stem and important cranial nerves.

This chapter describes a series of approaches which the author has found helpful over the years in general neurosurgical practice, and while it is likely that most neurosurgeons will have occasion to use most of these exposures only rarely, several of them such as the extended anterior temporal approach to the anterior tentorial hiatus, and the combined supra- and infratentorial approach to the upper clivus, give remarkably good access for a variety of conditions, and may therefore be considered of unusual practical value.

Pre-operative Management

General

Any approach to the tentorial hiatus, carrying as it does the hazard to perfusion of the upper brain stem, may result in a patient whose level of consciousness is reduced for many days. An adequate state of hydration must therefore be ensured for all patients whose post-operative level of consciousness is likely to be impaired. Few patients in the neurosurgical ward are a greater anxiety than the comatose post-operative craniopharyngioma, who, while in the end making an excellent recovery, may for several weeks require external control of his internal environment, his fluid balance, his temperature regulation and his intracranial pressure. It is wise therefore, to ensure that the patient's haematocrit and haemoglobin levels are normal before operation, to place the patient on Dexamethasone in the standard dosage (4 mgs six hourly), for several days pre-operatively, and to ensure an adequate post-operative hydration either by intravenous or nasogastric route. As soon as IV feeding may be discontinued, the management of fluid balance problems is considerably eased. The gut is a comfortably selective filter.

Antibiotic Cover

The routine use of antibiotics is to be discouraged in general neurosurgical practice, but the author finds it useful nevertheless to place all patients for craniotomy on Flucloxacillin, an antibiotic to which Staph. Epidermis is notably sensitive. Casual infections in the authors clinic over the years have almost invariably been with this troublesome organism, borne probably on the patients own skin, and the use of 2-3 days of Flucloxacillin pre-operatively and 3 or 4 days post-operatively, has virtually abolished wound infection. Doubtless as the hospital population of bacteria changes of course, added hazards may appear, and under no circumstances is there any substitute for careful aseptic surgery. The use of Flucloxacillin does not substitute for asepsis, it merely supplements as a safeguard against contamination from the patients own skin, complete sterilization of which is impossible.

Anaesthesia

The approaches described in this chapter are invariably performed under endotracheal general anaesthesia. In the authors clinic, this is usually induced with methohexital or thiopentone, the initial respiratory paralysis being achieved by succinyl choline, and the anaesthetic then continued with Halothane, Nitrous Oxide and Oxygen, or Halothane and Oxygen alone, continuing muscular paralysis being provided by D-tubo-curarine. In the recumbent or park-bench position, arterial hypotension down to mean arterial pressure levels of around 60-70 mm Mercury is entirely safe and of great value in the resection of troublesome vascular tumours, such as the clivus meningiomas. Where the patient has been placed in the seated position, as for the subtentorial approach to the posterior tentorial hiatus, then arterial hypotension is undesirable, and the patients blood pressure is carefully maintained with a mean in the region of 100 mms Mercury. It is the authors practice to reverse respiration and to raise the arterial BP to approximately the patients normal, before closure of the dura. This enables the degree of post-operative swelling to be assessed from the phase of increased arterial CO_2 tension before the patient breathes, and assurance of adequate haemostasis at normal arterial pressure is obtained.

The Use of c.s.f. Drainage

For the lateral approaches to the tentorial hiatus with the patient in the park bench position, lumbar drainage is frequently of value. The drain may be placed pre-operatively, and opened as the dura is prepared for incision. The drainage should be discontinued as haemostasis is proceeeding at the end of the procedure.

Tumours in the tentorial hiatus are frequently associated with hydro-cephalus. Preliminary ventriculo-peritoneal or ventriculo-atrial shunting procedures may therefore be considered and in some instances it will be found that these have been performed elsewhere, the major tumour itself, clivus meningioma for example, having been deemed inoperable. The advantages of preliminary shunt placement are of course that the patient's condition, if parlous, may be considerably improved before the major operation proceeds, but the notable disadvantage is that the tremendous relaxation provided by per-operative drainage of the c.s.f. spaces is no longer available. Except in cases whose clinical condition is truly critical, where urgent drainage of the ventricular system for more than a few days is required before definitive surgery, the author does not recommend prior ventricular shunting procedures. In the supra- and infratentorial approach to pineal tumours, or in the approach to any mass in the tentorial hiatus with gross hydrocephalus, continuous ventricular drainage may be of value. With the increased use of steroids (Dexamethasone in standard dosages), the necessity for continuous ventricular drainage post-operatively is now much less. Ventricular drainage may be used throughout the procedure, but in the author's practice it is rarely maintained post-operatively for more than a day or two. One of the salient advantages of the combined supra- and infratentorial approach is that the complete tentorial division, which removes the tentorial hiatus as a focus for post-operative cone, means that the decompression alone is usually sufficient to deal with post-operative swelling and continuous c.s.f. drainage is not required.

The Anterior Temporal Approach

This is undoubtedly the simplest approach to the anterior part of the
tentorial hiatus.

The practicability of approaching the upper part of the tentorial hiatus along
the sphenoidal wing was shown by Yaşargil (1976) in relation to aneurysms of
the top of the basilar artery, for which it is suitable in experienced hands. It is
however, a relatively constricted approach, unsuitable for extensive exposure,
and can be enlarged only if care is taken in the design of the approach to turn a
scalp and bone flap sufficiently large to enable the surgeon to move back into the
middle temporal region (see extended anterior temporal approach with temporal
lobectomy). In the true sphenoidal wing approach the flap turned is the same as
that for anterior circle aneurysms, running from the middle or lateral part of the
forehead, around the outer end of the sphenoidal wing, and down to in front of
the tragus, the scalp flap being turned downwards and forwards, and a small
bone flap cut through three or four burr holes including a double (spectacle) burr
hole across the sphenoidal wing, and broken down into the anterior temporal
fossa (Fig. 1). The dura should be opened round the outer end of the sphenoidal
wing, and the surgeon dissects first down the wing, to open the arachnoid over
the internal carotid artery. The inner end of the sylvian fissure may then be
dissected, together with the deep middle cerebral vein joining the spheno-
parietal or cavernous sinus, lateral to the internal carotid, if it exists, and such
other branches of the middle cerebral venous system, as may be necessary to
enable downward retraction of the tip of the temporal lobe and an extended
opening of the sylvian fissure, carrying the surgeon backwards along and lateral
to the internal carotid and posterior communicating arteries, with the third
nerve and edge of the tentorium below. Rosenthal's vein may be identified in
arachnoid lateral to the brain stem but frequently is retracted with the temporal
lobe. The posterior communicating artery is followed to its junction with the
posterior cerebral artery, and the surgeon then works medially to the anterior
part of the tentorial hiatus, and the top of the basilar artery. Where this
approach is to be used for basilar aneurysms, double self-retaining retraction will
usually be necessary, and it will usually be found that some damage to the
superior temporal gyrus, particularly in its deeper part, has been made by the
pressure of the retractor holding down the anterior temporal lobe. Of greater
significance is the fact that the subfrontal retraction as it moves backwards to
elevate the hemisphere and display the posterior communicating artery, may
very well occasion retractor pressure on the middle cerebral in its proximal
portion. Such retractor pressure has been known since Penfield's day as a major
cause of hemiparesis after temporal lobectomy, and must be most carefully
avoided.

As Yaşargil himself has pointed out, the main disadvantage to the anterior
temporal approach to the basilar bifurcation is its technical difficulty, requiring
considerable experience and training with the operating microscope and microsurgical techniques. Drake's view (1979) is that the approach can be narrow and
confining, though ideal for aneurysms with small necks lying just above or below
the dorsum sellae, and pointing forward or upward.

In the author's view, while this restricted approach may be adequate for exposure of upward and forward pointing aneurysms of the terminal basilar artery, it is too constricting for dealing with neoplasms in the tentorial hiatus, or on the top of the dorsum sellae, and the author would prefer the use of the extended anterior temporal approach, (vide infra) with limited temporal lobectomy.

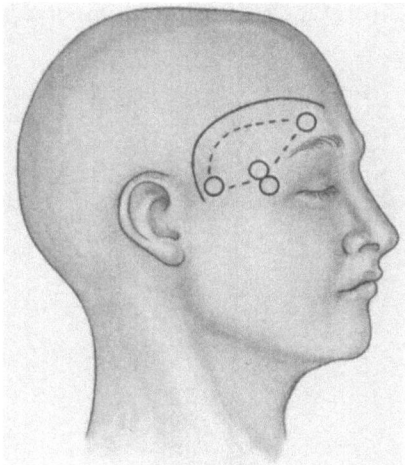

Fig. 1. Scalp and bone flap for the anterior temporal approach along the sphenoidal wing

The closure of this approach is routine for a standard craniotomy, careful closure of the dura with interrupted black silk sutures and the replacement of the bone flap with a perforating "Poppen" stitch, and a careful muscle closure. It is the author's uniform practice to employ subgaleal suction drainage for 48 hours post-operatively, except where extensive dural defects have been left behind, and the use of such drains is recommended in this procedure.

The Extended Anterior Temporal Approach with Anterior Temporal Lobectomy

This is the approach now used by the author for many terminal basilar aneurysms, and for the resection of tumours within the anterior part of the tentorial hiatus, such as meningioma of the dorsum sellae or posterior suprasellar region, and craniopharyngioma.

The majority of craniopharyngiomas in the author's personal series of over sixty adult cases, have presented in the floor of the third ventricle, occupying the suprasellar and interpeduncular cisterns, and embraced by the branches of the posterior communicating and choroidal arteries to the thalamus and mamillary bodies. The postero-inferior presenting portion of such tumours lies free in the interpeduncular cistern and gives a considerable quadrant of the mass available for early excision, albeit through an extremely limited access between the branches of the posterior communicating artery, or below the posterior communicating artery itself. The appropriate approach therefore is frequently the extended temporal approach to the tentorial hiatus.

With the advent of the operating microscope, this procedure has increasingly become the approach of choice. An extended sphenoidal wing approach is used, a moderately sized fronto-temporal flap being turned from the middle of the eyebrow, just below the superior temporal line to above the ear, and turning down in front of the pinna (Fig. 2). A fronto-temporal bone flap cut across the

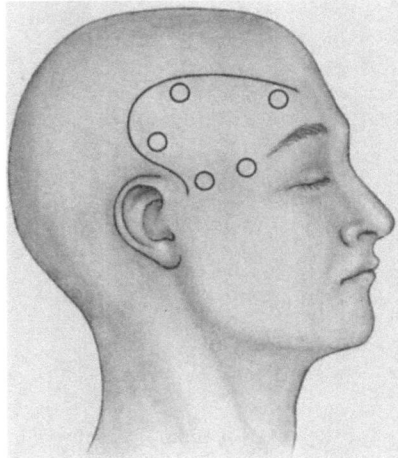

Fig. 2. Position of scalp and bone flap for the extended anterior temporal approach with limited temporal lobectomy

sphenoidal wing is broken down into the anterior temporal fossa. The anterior part of the temporal fossa is then rongeured away together with the outer end of the sphenoidal wing, and the dura opened across the sylvian fissure so that access to the subfrontal and anterior temporal region is assured. The next step is a small resection of the anterior two centimetres of the temporal lobe, with division of the polar temporal veins so that the subfrontal region is laid into continuity with the anterior of the temporal fossa. Under the operating microscope, the inner end of the sylvian fissure can then be opened, the carotid artery and the optic nerve defined, and dissection pursued behind the carotid artery, along the tentorial edge. Removal of the uncus by secondary suction will give access to the tentorial hiatus and interpeduncular fossa. At this stage, the presenting lower pole of a craniopharyngioma for example (Fig. 3), will be evident in the interpeduncular cistern, and immediately lateral to it and in their own separate arachnoid, the posterior communicating artery, its thalamo-perforating branches and the third nerve. With the division of arachnoid in the interpeduncular fossa, the top of the basilar artery and its branches may be defined (Fig. 4).

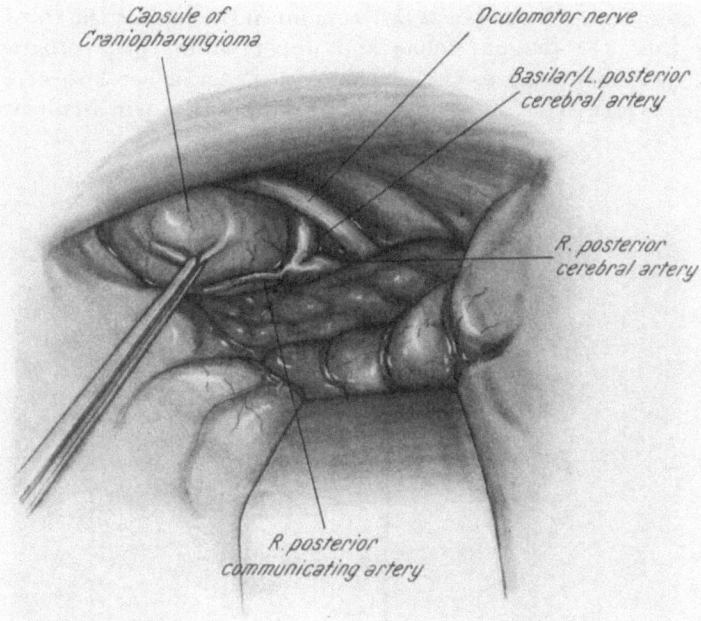

Fig. 3. Exposure of the capsule of a craniopharyngioma by the extended anterior temporal approach to the tentorial hiatus, combined with a small temporal lobectomy. The arachnoid covering of craniopharyngioma in the tentorial hiatus is held in the forceps for incision

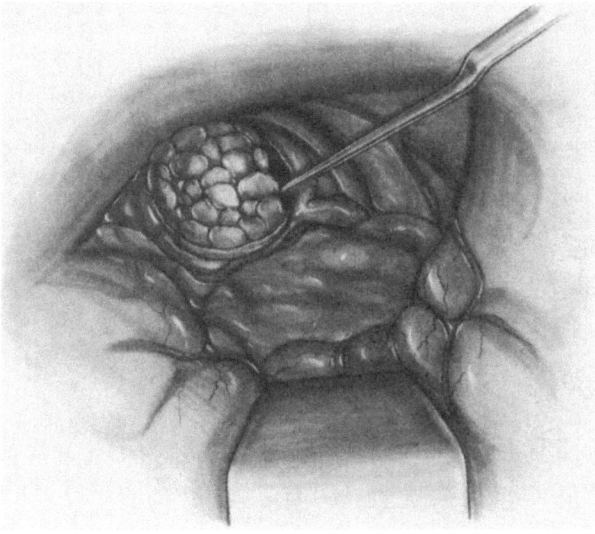

Fig. 4. The exposure of craniopharyngioma continues. The tumour has now been freed from its arachnoid coverings for dissection

The postero-inferior portion of any tumour in the base of the third ventricle, or arising from the dorsum sellae and upper clivus, may progressively be mobilised, its attachment to the basilar and posterior cerebral arteries being defined and divided. The full radiological work up is shown in an illustrative case

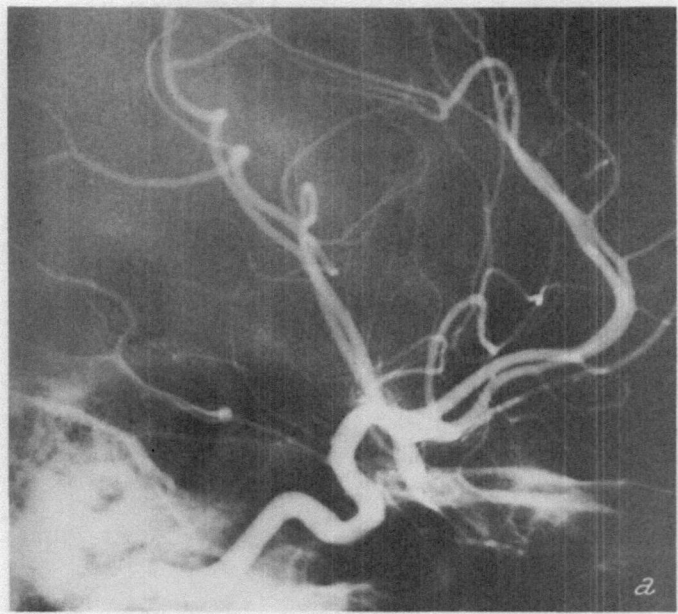

Fig. 5. A case of intrinsic craniopharyngioma. Right and left lateral carotid arteriograms (a and b) and vertebral arteriography (c) display the great stretching of the posterior communicating vessels with separation and curvature of the thalamo-perforating and choroidal arteries. Lateral filling (d) and brow-up (e) views of the air encephalogram confirm the large mass, extending from the interpeduncular cistern to the interthalamic connexus and the Foramen of Monro. Post-operative lateral air encephalogram (f) shows successful excision of the mass with communication between the interpeduncular fossa and the third ventricle on the filling films. The boy, a twelve year old, made an uninterrupted recovery, but had of course diabetes insipidus, requiring nasal DDAVP. There was no other neurological defect

in Fig. 5. Aneurysms of the upper part of the basilar artery are extensively exposed (Figs. 6 and 7). Illustrative cases are demonstrated in Figs. 8 and 9. The utility of the approach is clear in the case of separated multiple aneurysms (Fig. 9).

The extended temporal approach is closed in a manner similar to the straight forward anterior temporal approach, and once again it is appropriate to apply continuous suction drainage in the subgaleal space for some 48 hours.

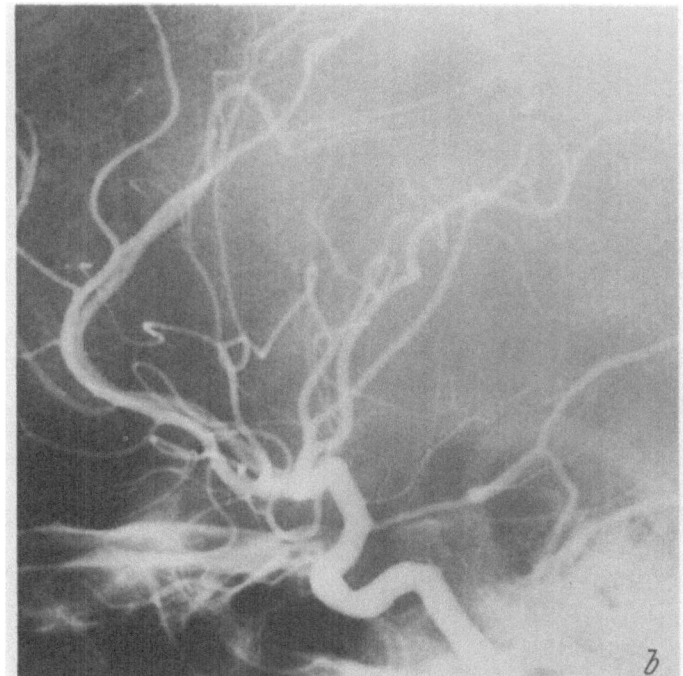

Fig. 5 b

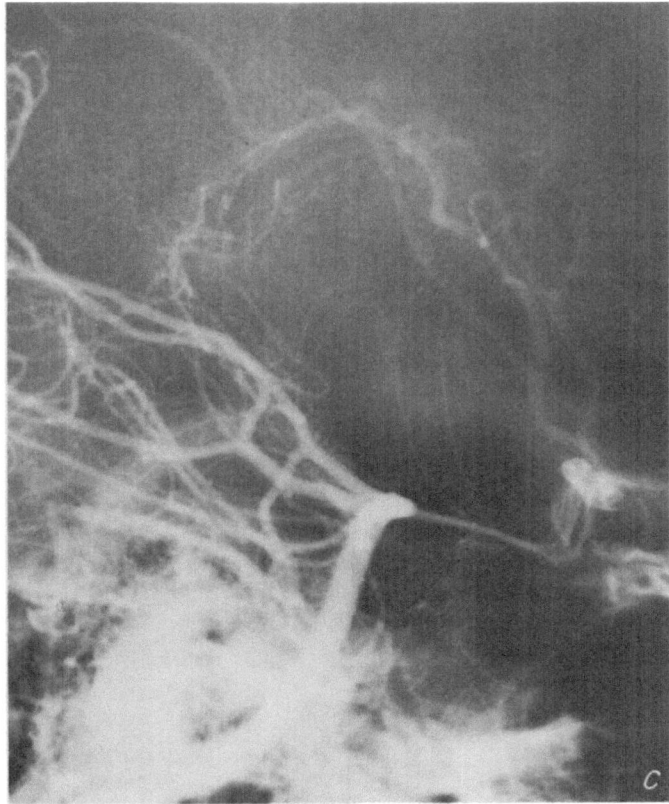

Fig. 5 c

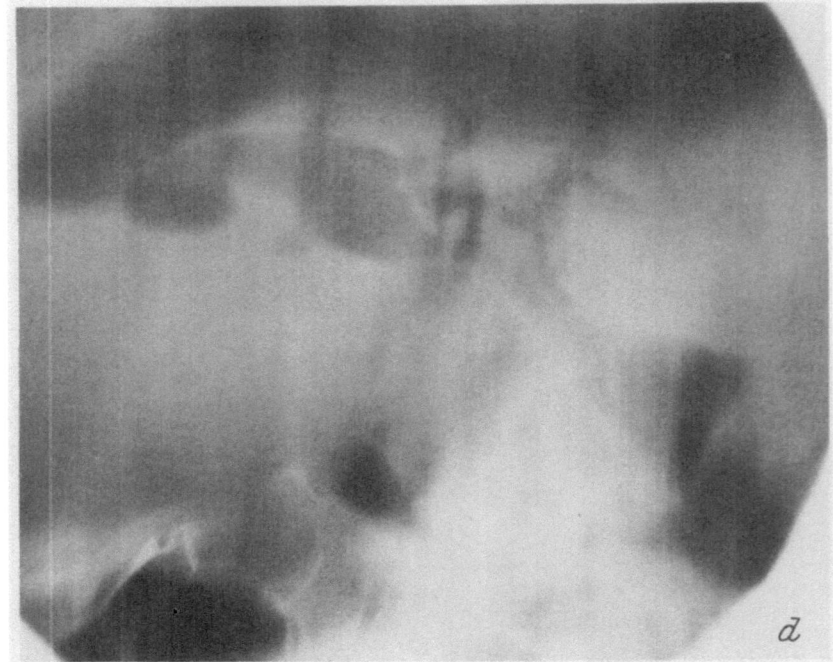

Fig. 5 d

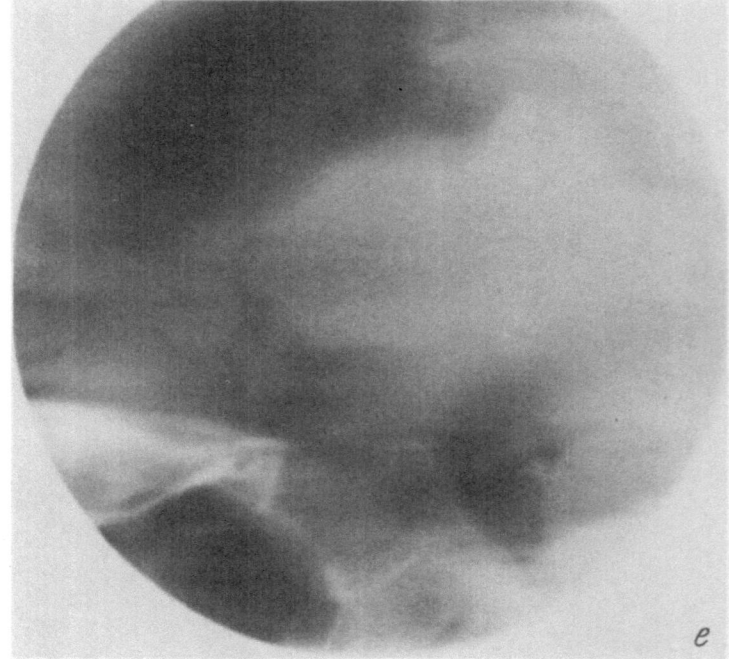

Fig. 5 e

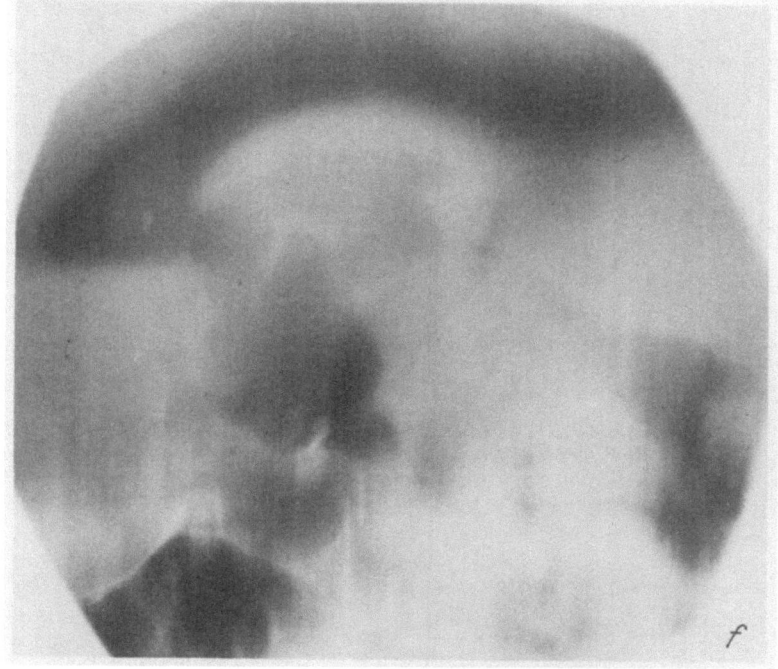

Fig. 5 f

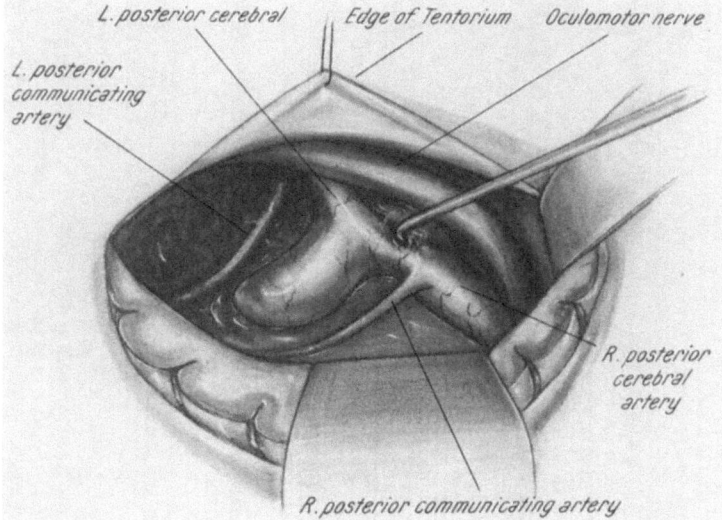

Fig. 6. The dissection of an anteriorly pointing large basilar aneurysm. The retractor defines the posteriorly placed perforators from the proximal basilar artery by retraction of the first part of posterior cerebral on the right side. The two posterior communicating arteries are visible

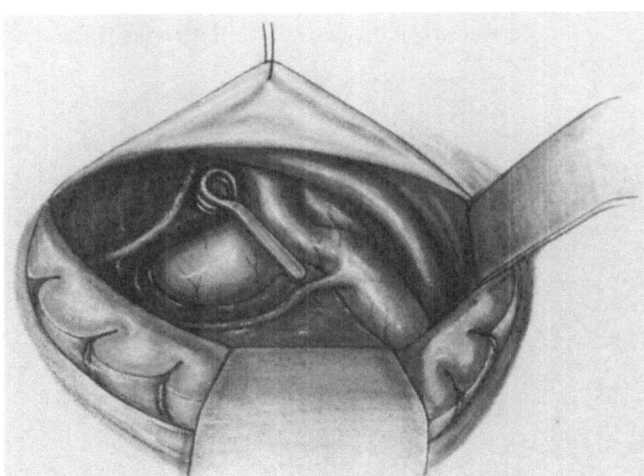

Fig. 7. Diagram to show the application of a clip to terminal basilar aneurysm by the described technique using a small anterior temporal lobectomy. The extent of visualization of both posterior cerebral arteries is clear, the basilar trunk is scarcely visible, passing downwards behind the arachnoid. The diagram is drawn from operative video tape

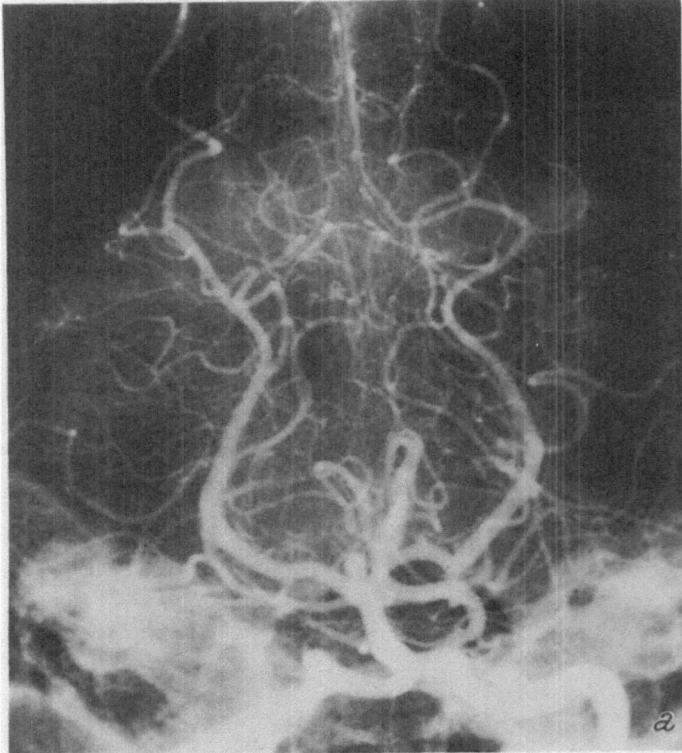

Fig. 8. A small basilar tip aneurysm in a young woman. The V shaping of the take-off of posterior cerebrals favoured in anterior approach. AP and lateral pre (a and b) and post operative films (c and d) show the aneurysm and its occlusion

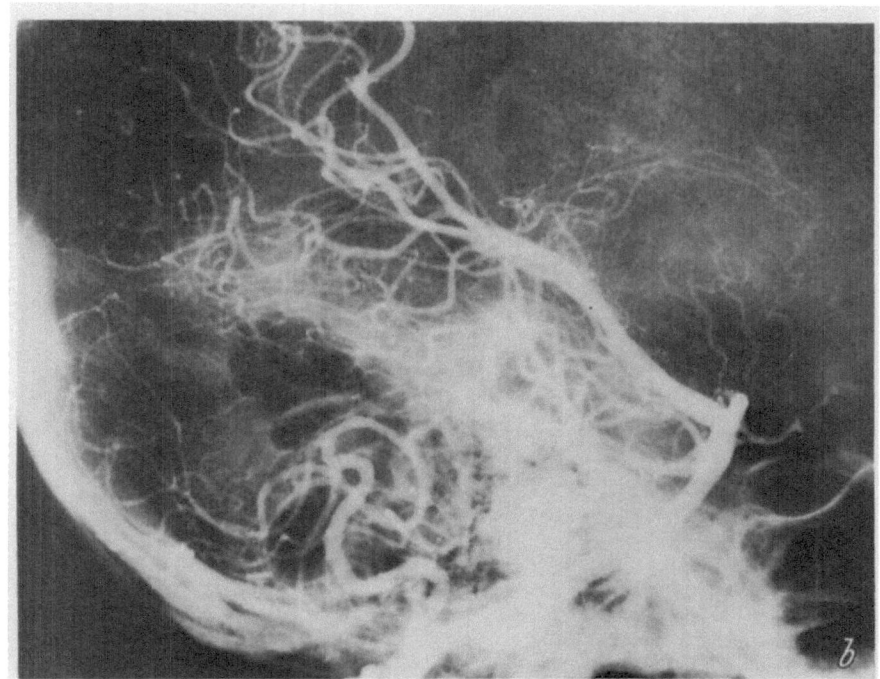

Fig. 8 b

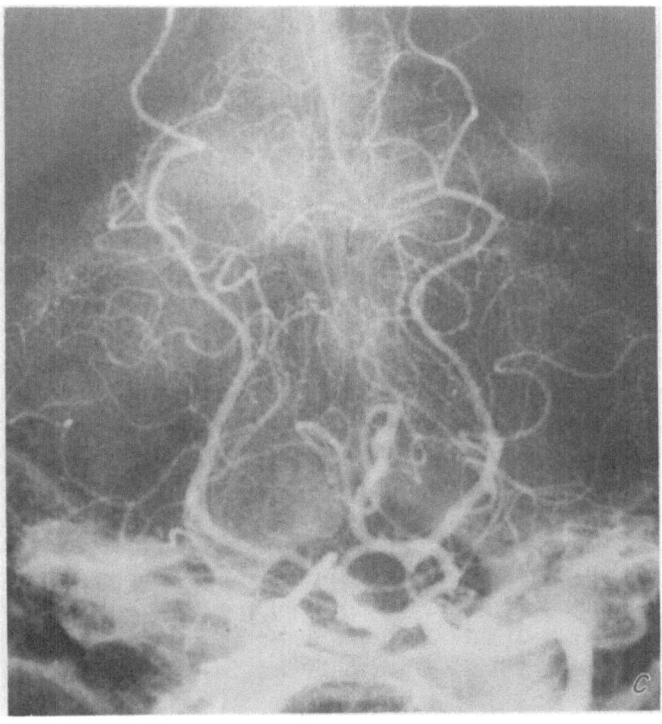

Fig. 8 c

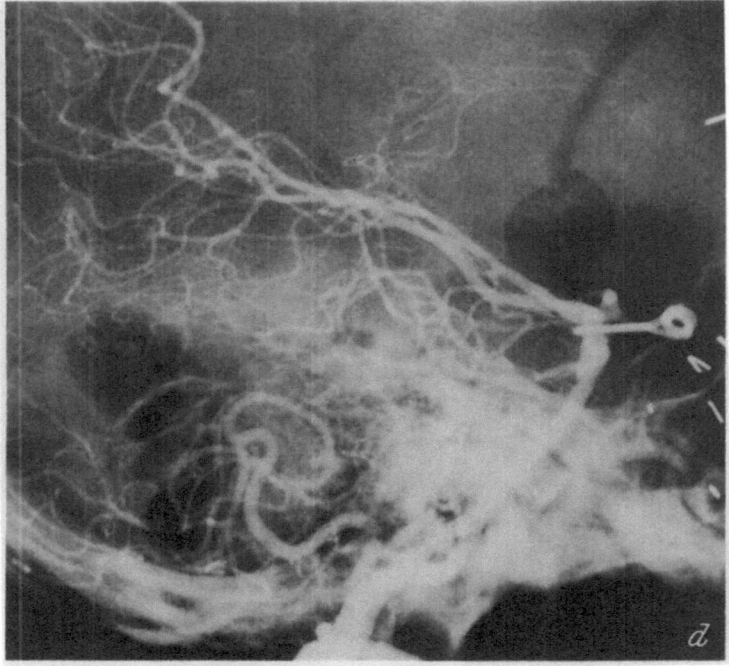

Fig. 8 d

The Subtemporal Approach to the Tentorial Hiatus

This approach has been designed and popularised by Charles Drake (1965), principally in relation to aneurysms of the upper part of the basilar artery. It is therefore an alternative approach to the sphenoidal wing approach recommended by Yaşargil in relation to these aneurysms, but the indications for the two approaches are perhaps a little different. Thus, from the anterior temporal or sphenoidal wing approach, particularly if combined with the extended temporal approach including a small temporal lobectomy, the view of the surgeon twoards the contralateral posterior cerebral artery is considerably better than that by the classical Drake subtemporal approach across the floor of the middle fossa. On the other hand, the view of the sheaf of perforating vessels running behind an aneurysm of the basilar bifurcation into the interpeduncular fossa and brain stem, is considerably better by the true lateral approach. In many ways, provided sacrifice of the anterior inch or so of the temporal pole is not considered unacceptable, the extended anterior temporal approach provides the benefits of both the sphenoidal wing and lateral subtemporal approach.

For the true lateral subtemporal approach, the patient is positioned on his side with the neck slightly flexed downwards and careful support of the underlying prominences. A pad should be placed in the axilla, pads under the underlying arm and pads under the underlying lateral popliteal nerve. Drake has

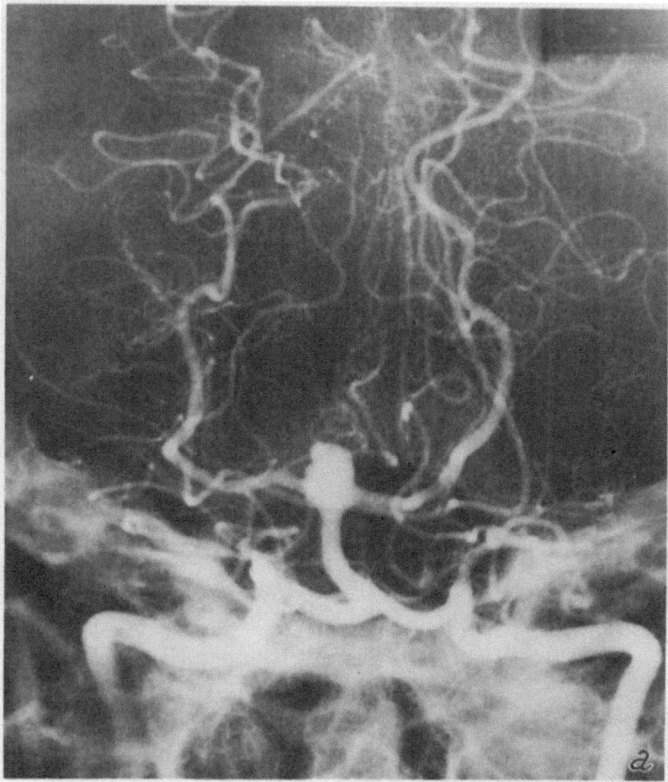

Fig. 9. AP (a) and lateral (b) vertebral arteriography and an oblique film of a right carotid arteriogram (c) of the same patient, a 36-year-old woman. The carotid angiogram indicated the presence of a small anterior communicating artery aneurysm, whose anatomy was difficult to define, even in multiple projections, but it was thought that the larger basilar aneurysm had bled. The lesion was attacked from anteriorly, using a small anterior temporal lobectomy to occlude the basilar aneurysm, which had a broad base. Two clips were required. The small anterior communicating aneurysm had in fact bled and was satisfactorily occluded at the same time. Post-operative views show AP and lateral vertebral arteriography (d and e), and slightly oblique AP view of the carotid circulation (f)

recommended either a small curved incision in front of the ear, or a linear incision, as for the standard Frazier approach to the Gasserian ganglion, but most less experienced surgeons will prefer a straight forward mid temporal flap, turned down above the ear, under which is fashioned a straight forward four burr hole flap, carried right down to the floor of the temporal fossa. It is wise in the pre-operative work up to identify the position of Labbés vein, although it may be impossible to secure adequate retraction without considerable danger to this vessel. The dura is opened in a U shaped incision based superiorly with re-entrant incisions below, the dural edges held back, and if the lower end of the

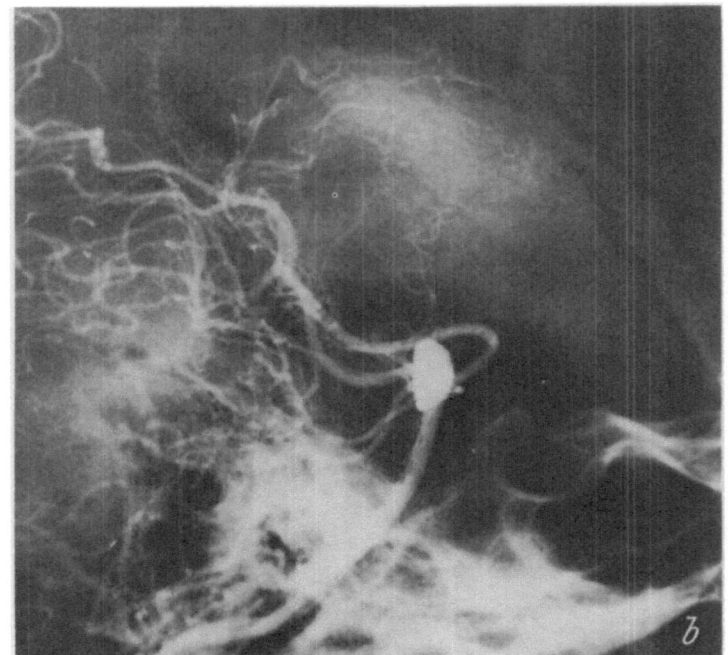

Fig. 9 b

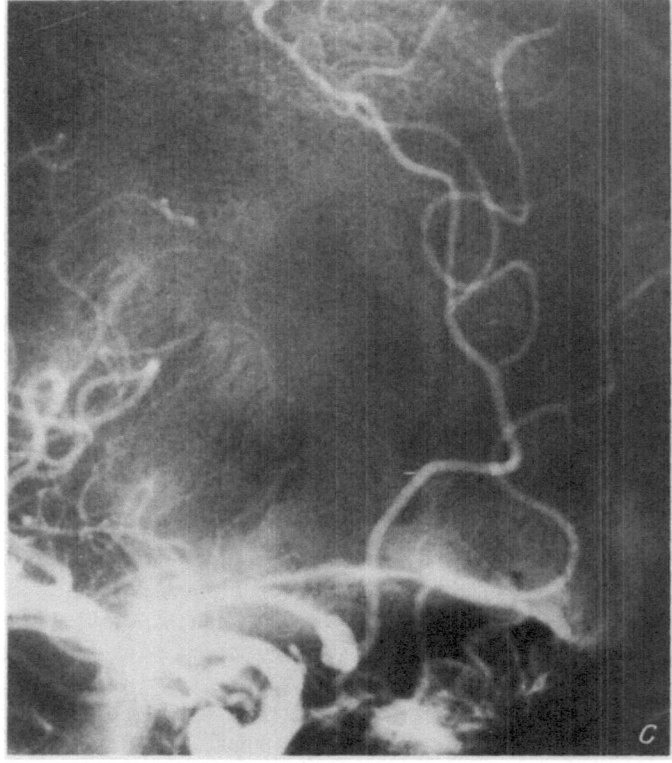

Fig. 9 c

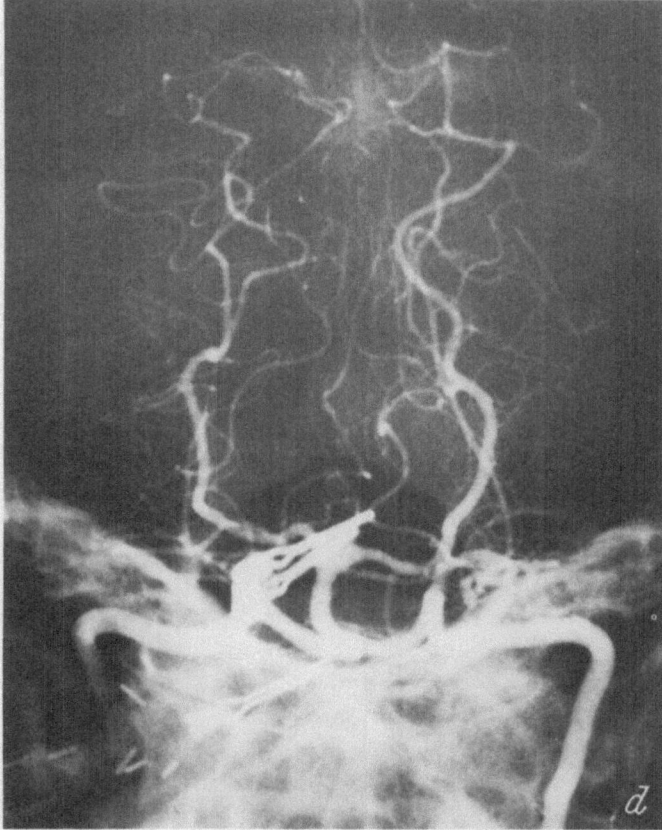

Fig. 9 d

flap has been adequately sited, dissection pursued straight across the floor of the temporal fossa, towards the tentorial hiatus. A number of veins crossing from the temporal lobe to the floor of the fossa may be encountered and must be divided, but as far as possible, Drake has recommended that Labbés vein be preserved. Self retaining retraction of the Yaşargil type is employed with the retractor post sited superiorly, and retraction may be deep and occasionally fairly heavy on the temporal lobe, particularly if there is brain swelling associated with recent subarachnoid haemorrhage. It is necessary therefore to cover the exposed brain carefully with lintine and to remove this lintine at the close by lavage rather than simply dragging it off the underlying brain. The self retaining retraction should approach the tentorial hiatus, and as Drake has pointed out, it may then be a help to place a suture through the free edge of the tentorium avoiding the fourth nerve, and anchor this down to the floor of the temporal fossa, thus counteracting the upward slope of the medial part of the tentorium and improving the access to the hiatus. The structures which must be

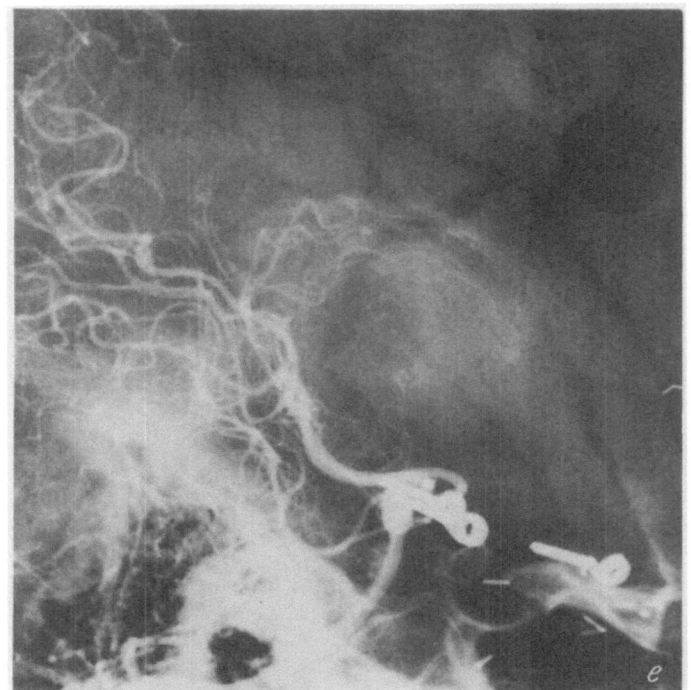

Fig. 9 e

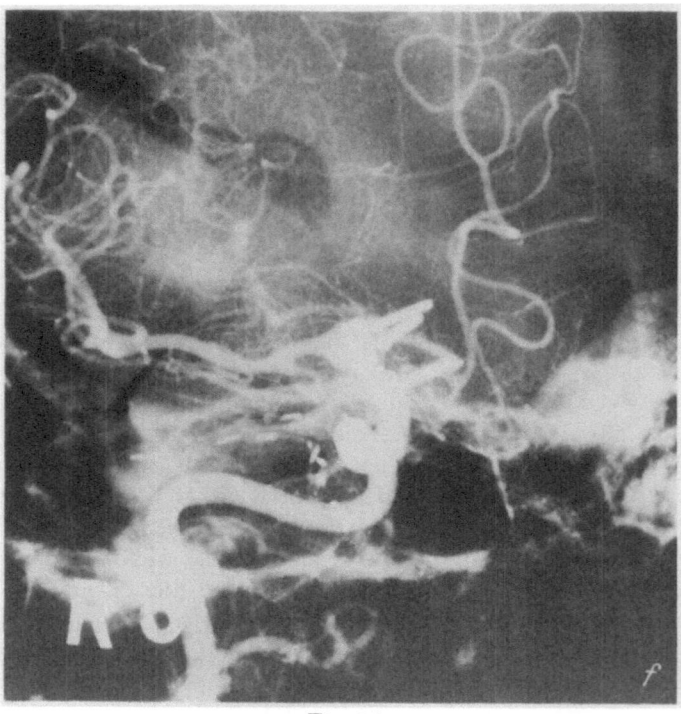

Fig. 9 f

avoided as the hiatus is approached are of course the posterior communicating artery and the third nerve. Dissection under the operating microscope however, usually enables the arachnoid to be opened by sharp dissection carefully with these structures visualised through the intact arachnoid, and appropriately avoided. It must be admitted that a partial third nerve palsy is not an infrequent complication of this approach, but that the nerve invariably recovers.

This approach carries the authority of the world's most experienced posterior circulation surgeon, and must therefore be regarded as adequate for the majority of aneurysms at the upper end of the basilar artery.

Drake himself has indicated that resection of the temporal lobe has never been necessary in his series of basilar tip aneurysms, and who is to argue with a surgeon who now has operated on over 600 of the lesions. Regrettably however, our problem is not the surgeon who has operated on over 600 basilar aneurysms, but the surgeon who operates on only a few. It will be apparent therefore that approach to the upper part of the basilar artery demands room, and in this author's contention, that room may be most readily acquired by sacrifice of a portion of the non-dominant temporal lobe.

Where extended access to a tumour, as for example a meningioma of the upper dorsum sellae, is required, the approach is somewhat inadequate. While brain resection is to be regretted if avoidable, brain resection is preferable to extensive brain necrosis and post-operative swelling induced by excessive retraction, and this must always be considered when the mid temporal approach is used for extended exposure of the lateral aspect of the tentorial hiatus.

Closure is straight forward. The dura is repaired with interrupted black silk sutures, the bone flap replaced with a single perforating stitch and multiple pericranial sutures, and the scalp closed in two layers with suction drainage.

From these three approaches to the anterior and lateral portion of the tentorial hiatus, it will be evident that personal preference plays a great role. Thus, notable technical surgeons such as Drake and Yaşargil, have differed in their recommended approach to the upper basilar artery, each finding the approach recommended by the other somewhat confining and less satisfactory than their own preferred technique. The lessons are clear, a surgeon is comfortable with the technique to which he is accustomed, and the less experienced surgeon should consider carefully the benefits of a relaxed and adequate exposure, and perhaps avoid attempts to emulate too closely, the surgical maestro.

The Combined Supra- and Infratentorial Approach to the Lateral Aspect of the Tentorial Hiatus

There is no approach which gives as extensive an exposure of the clivus from the posterior clinoids to the foramen magnum as this combined supra- and infratentorial exposure, and it is of particular use therefore in the approach to clivus meningiomas, large or difficult aneurysms of the basilar artery anywhere over its entire length, or tumours with extensive spread in posterior and middle fossas, such as cholesteatoma of the tentorial hiatus (Derome and Guiot 1979). Its use in the author's hands has been largely confined to these three conditions, clivus and apical petrous tumours, meningioma, paragrasserian tumours or clivus chordoma, (fifteen cases), difficult or complex upper basilar aneurysms, eight cases; and cholesteatomas of the posterior fossa tentorial hiatus and supratentorial region, six cases. The difficulty of approach to such lesions has often been emphasised (Davis and Martin 1939, Love and Walkman 1942, Ver Brugghen 1952, Krayenbühl and Yaşargil 1975). The author has also used this approach in angiomas of the upper medial cerebellum or vermis (3 cases) or on the superior brainstem itself (2 cases). Illustrative examples are shown in Figs. 13 to 19.

Essential Preliminary Investigations

It is wise in the planning of this approach to carry out complete angiography. This should include carefully taken venous phases, and the competence of both lateral sinuses should be assured. It may be difficult to ascertain that crossover occurs at the torcular Herophili between the two lateral sinuses, but a reasonable inference may be made if venous blood from both hemispheres appears in each lateral sinus (Fig. 10). Where one lateral sinus is dominant, and particularly if the other is absent, then division of the lateral sinus in this approach is probably unwise. With these reservations however, the author has divided the lateral sinus on either side without venous infarction, save in one case, a complex clivus meningioma, already attacked elsewhere, with an anomalous posterior circulation on the same side, the posterior cerebral vessels being partly embedded in the upper part of the tumour, and, being double, part coming from the basilar artery, and part from the carotid by an enlarged posterior communicating artery. However, division of the large, left lateral sinus for access in this case was associated with the development a few hours after the close of a long and difficult operation, of haemorrhagic infarction in the post temporo-occipital region on the left, with disastrous results for the patient. Although the lateral sinuses appeared competent, the left was much larger in this instance, and the possibility must at least be admitted that division of the lateral sinus occasioned a venous infarct. The author would not therefore recommend division of the left lateral sinus where this is very much the larger of the two, and the hemispheral dominance is left sided.

Positioning the Patient

For this approach, the patient is best placed in the park bench position (Fig. 11) with a little less rotation than would be necessary to bring the petrous face vertical, as for example in the resection of an acoustic neuroma. It is also wise to have the head approximately horizontal, rather than laterally flexed towards the inferior shoulder as for an upper posterior fossa approach, since the greater part of the exposure of the upper posterior fossa in the combined supra- and infratentorial approach is achieved by the division of the tentorium.

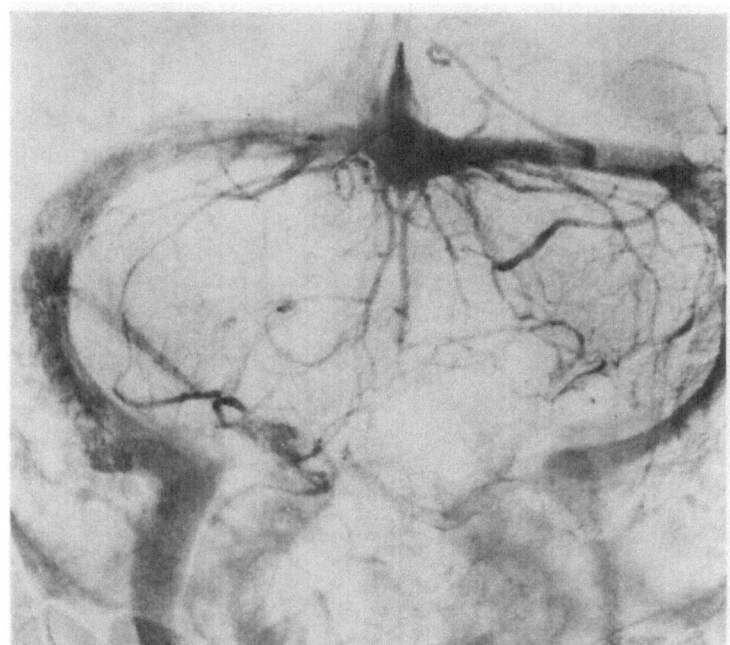

Fig. 10. Subtraction views of the venous phases of a vertebral arteriogram, showing good filling of both lateral sinuses. This type of film, or a comparable film from bilateral carotid arteriography, is essential before division of one lateral sinus is undertaken

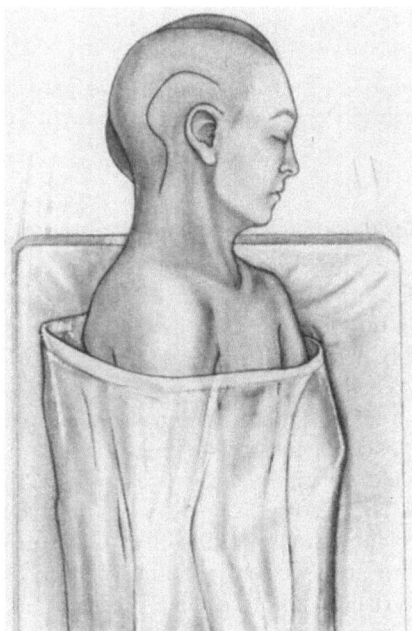

Fig. 11. Skin incision and position of the patient for the combined supra- and infra-tentorial approach to the tentorial hiatus

The Incision

The incision combines a mid-temporal supratentorial approach with a lateral posterior fossa approach, and the incision therefore is a mixture of the two ending up as a question mark form, the posteriorly directed supratentorial portion enabling reflection of the sinuous posterior limb of the infratentorial portion, and adequate posterior extension of the exposure of the bone in the region of the lateral sinus. The curved supratentorial component enables the

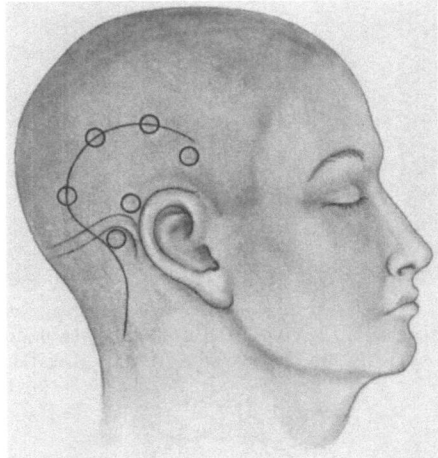

Fig. 12. Incision and situation of burr holes for the combined supra- and infratentorial approach to the lateral aspect of the tentorial hiatus

scalp flap to be turned down across the pinna, and a small supratentorial bone flap to be centered on the middle of the temporal muscle (Fig. 12). The supratentorial bone flap may be extended across the lateral sinus as is shown in the diagram, but if the burr hole at the base of the petrous bone proves difficult to make, it is probably wise to turn the supratentorial flap separately, and fashion either a further small plaque excision of bone in the infratentorial compartment, or as is the author's common practice, a generous craniectomy in the upper part of the posterior fossa. The key burr hole in the making of this flap is the burr hole at the base of the petrous pyramid. With care, and the use of an instrument such as the Hall drill, it is usually possible to fashion this burr hole to expose the supratentorial dura and the infratentorial dura across the lateral sinus, close to its junction with the sigmoid. Care must be taken in the manufacture of this burr hole not to avulse the mastoid emissory vein from the junction of the sigmoid and lateral sinuses, as the bone is resected. If a portion of this vein can be left intact for coagulation, this is much easier to handle than a rent in the lateral sinus wall.

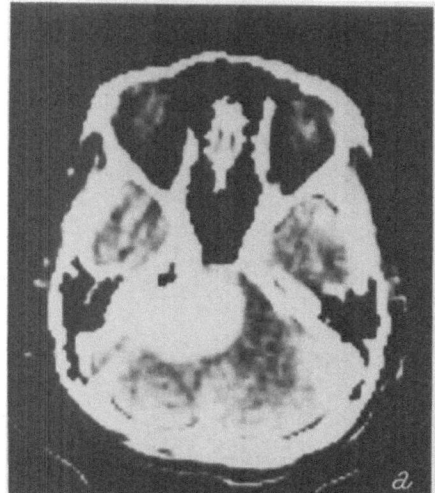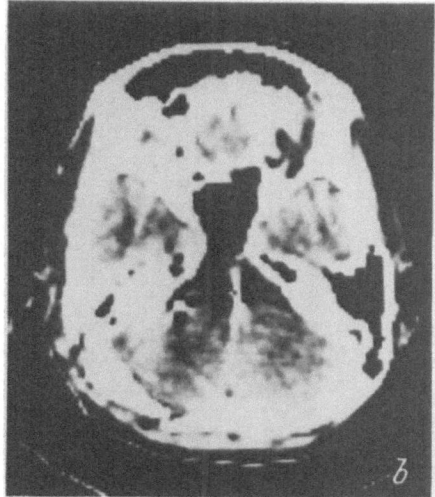

Fig. 13 a and b. Pre- and post-operative CT scans of a 47-year-old lady with a seven year history of gradually increasing deafness in the left ear, left sided trigeminal neuralgia, and increasing ataxia. Examination showed mild papilloedema, left sided cerebellar signs and slight ataxia, a reduced corneal reflex and sensory neural impairment of hearing on the left side

Post-operative CT scan shows that the mass has been successfully removed. The patient was completely deaf and had a complete sixth nerve palsy post-operatively, but seventh nerve and fifth nerve functions were completely preserved. The mass extended from the Foramen Magnum to the supratentorial compartment

From the preliminary angiography, the position of Labbés vein will have been identified. It is as a rule possible to preserve Labbés vein, particularly if, as is frequently the case, it enters the tentorium some way anterior to its final junction with the lateral sinus. It is then possible to divide the lateral sinus anterior to the entry point of Labbés vein, and to retract the vein with the the tentorial leaf on the subtemporal brain behind self retaining retractors. Labbés vein then goes with the hemisphere, drains to the torcula behind, and is preserved. Where Labbés vein enters very far anteriorly, it may be possible to divide the lateral sinus behind the entry point of Labbés vein, but the vein then passes across the exposure and is at continuous risk. This position of the vein is fortunately considerably less common than the other, but the vein itself has perforce been sacrificed in the course of the procedure on several occasions, as a result of being stretched and torn, fortunately without serious consequences in any case. The effort to preserve this important vein is worthwhile.

Opening the Dura

With the position of Labbés vein in mind, linear dural incisions are made along the base of the middle fossa and along the top of the posterior fossa, above the line of the sigmoid sinus with a further posterior fossa dural incision below

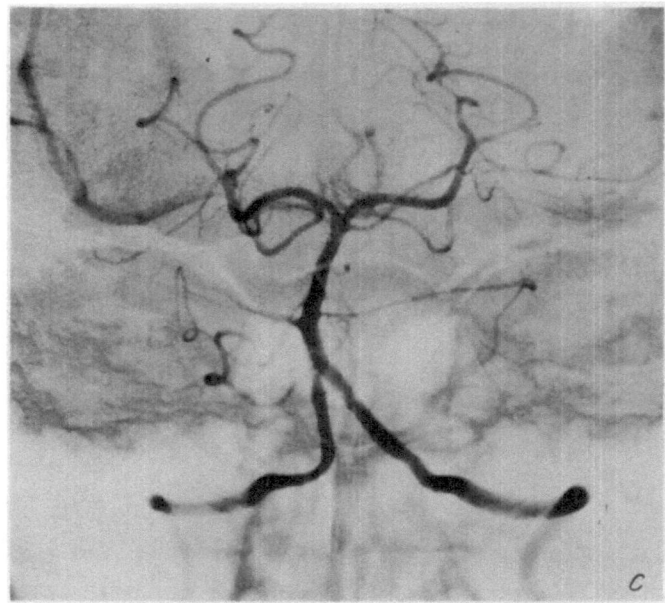

Fig. 13 c. AP vertebral arteriograms. The left vertebral and basilar arteries are displaced to the right and posteriorly, the left AIC, and to a lesser extent, the left superior cerebellar artery posteriorly and superiorly

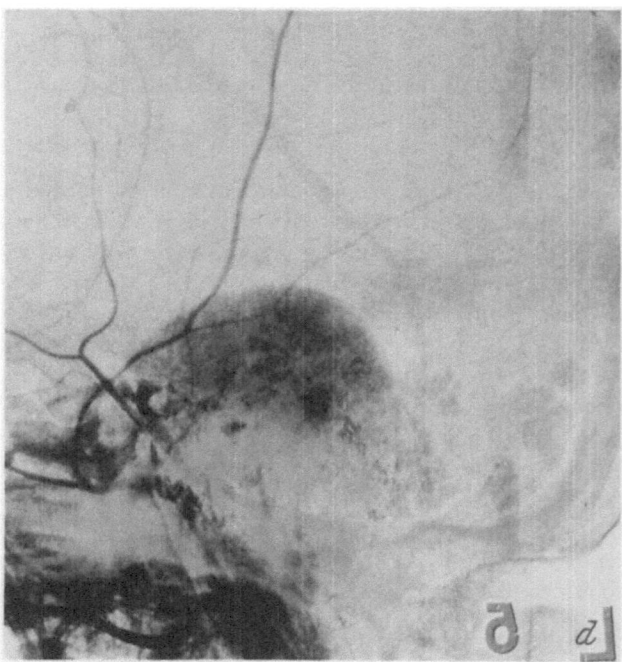

Fig. 13 d. A subtraction view of the lateral projection of an external carotid arteriogram. As usual with apical petrous and clivus tumours, the capillary circulation is mainly external in origin, together with meningeal branches from the petrous portion of the internal carotid artery, not seen on this film

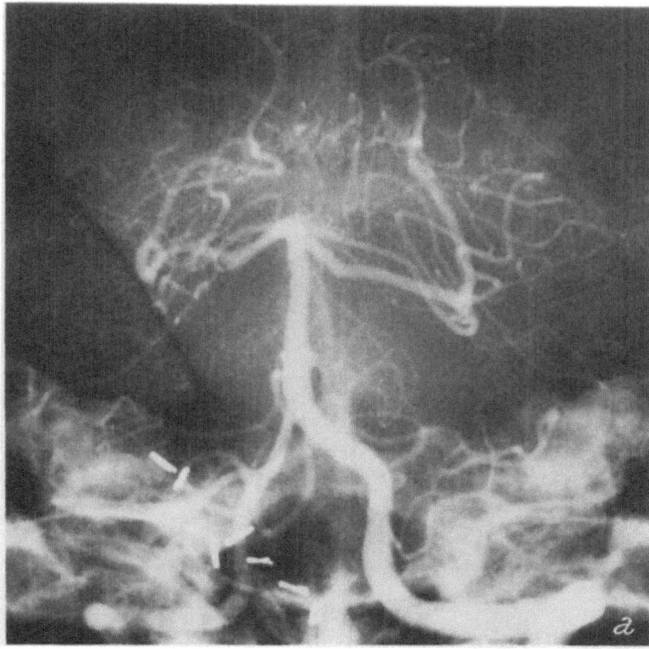

Fig. 14 a and b. AP and lateral vertebral arteriograms in a case of chordoma of the clivus. The silver clips indicate the previous right frontal exploration at the time when the tumour produced chiasmatic compression from a suprasellar extension. The posterior displacement of the basilar artery is visible, together with the downward displacement of AIC and the rather unusual sharp angulation of the origins of the two posterior cerebral arteries, indicating their close attachment to the upper part of the mass. The mass was successfully removed by combined supra- and infratentorial approach. Pre-operatively, the patient had a complete left sided cavernous sinus syndrome, with appreciable ataxia. The cavernous sinus syndrome was unchanged post-operatively, but the ataxia markedly improved

the sinus. White silk transfixion ligatures are placed through the tentorium, medial to the sinus, and brought out through the edges of the dural incisions, just above and just below the sinus (Fig. 18). These are firmly tied and the sinus divided between them. The tentorium may then be divided into the tentorial hiatus in the desired direction, and it is usually wise to carry this division as close to the edge of the petrous bone as possible (Fig. 19). The cerebellar veins enter the tentorium further back than this plane of division, and the only infra-tentorial vein which appears in the field is therefore the petrosal vein just lateral to the fifth nerve, high in the cerebello-pontine angle. Supratentorially, Labbés vein, having been retracted with the posterior dural flap, is protected from injury, and smaller bridging veins between the temporal lobe and the inferior aspect of the temporal fossa, the upper aspect of the petrous bone, may be divided without problem. Double self retaining retractors of the Yaşargil type

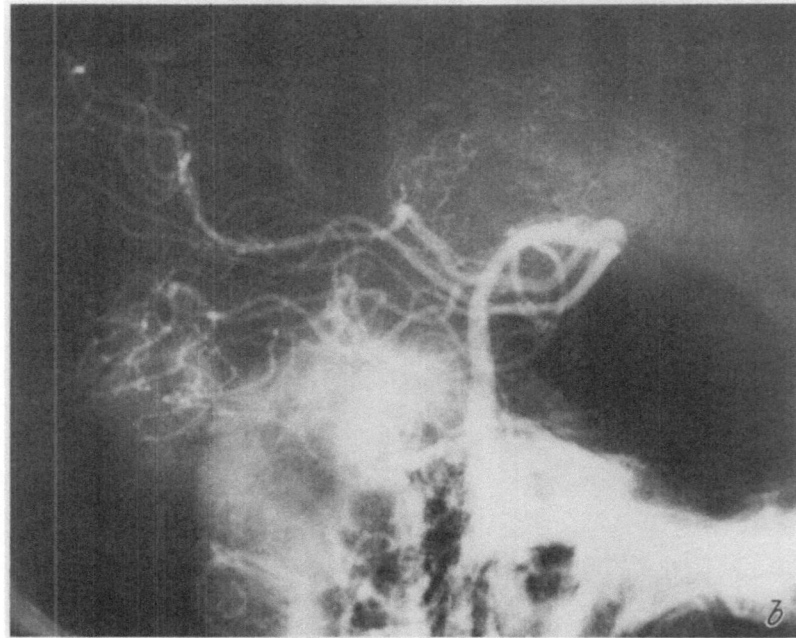

Fig. 14 b

skull mounted, have been uniformly used by the author in this approach, and it is quite surprising how little retraction of the cerebellum downwards and of the temporal lobe upwards is needed to enable the brain to open like a book, hinging on the tentorial edge. Under the microscope, the division of the arachnoid close to the tentorial edge, and of the medial part of the tentorium, may be carried out with preservation of the fourth nerve, and the detailed anatomy of the tentorial hiatus inspected. Of course, with a tentorial meningioma, or a clivus tumour, the tumour itself will usually have been uncovered by the time the medial part of the tentorium is reached, and it frequently proves impossible to dissect the fourth nerve out of the meningioma if it is involved within it, although a determined effort will usually result in sparing of the third cranial nerve, a more substantial and forgiving structure. It regenerates well.

Where the exposure is for an extensive cholesteatoma, then resection of the tumour will progressively decompress the mass, reveal the line of the brain stem, and the likely point of origin of the cranial nerves, which may then be followed through the cholesteatoma to the posterior aspect of the cavernous sinus. In the author's experience, the oculo-motor nerves, 3, 4 and 6, retain their identity quite well through cholesteatoma, but the 5th nerve has frequently been spread out in multiple parts, and has almost always been partially damaged in the resection. Fortunately, this has usually been heralded by some partial 5th nerve disability before operation, sometimes trigeminal neuralgia in the case of

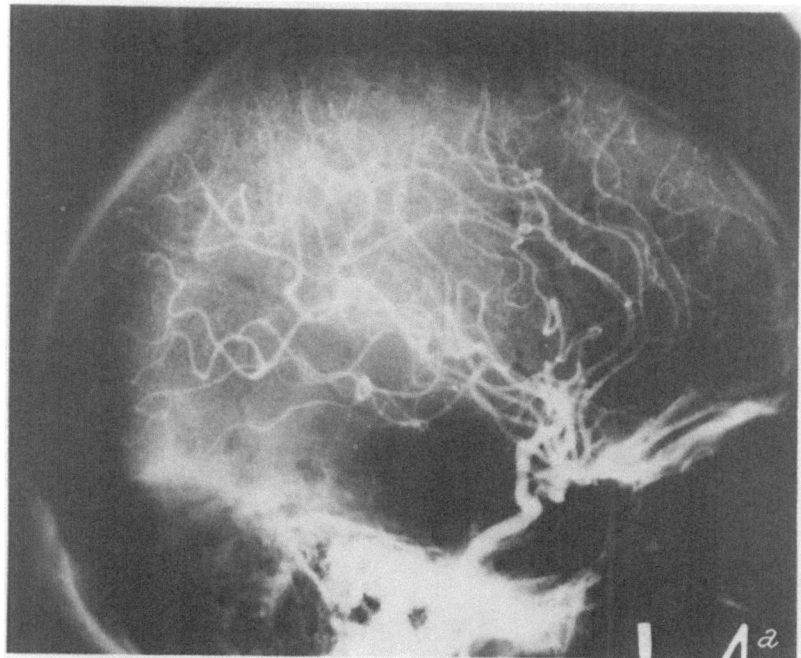

Fig. 15 a–d. A large middle and posterior fossa cholesteatoma in a 45-year-old lady. The arterial and venous phases of the carotid arteriogram (a and b) show gross swelling of the left temporal region, and indicate the position of Labbés vein. The AP and lateral vertebral arteriograms (c and d) show the enormous extension into the posterior fossa with gross elevation of the posterior cerebral and superior cerebellar arteries, separation spreading of the thalamo-perforating vessels and downward placement of the lower posterior fossa branches of the basilar. The lesion was attacked by a left sided combined supra and infratentorial approach and successfully excised

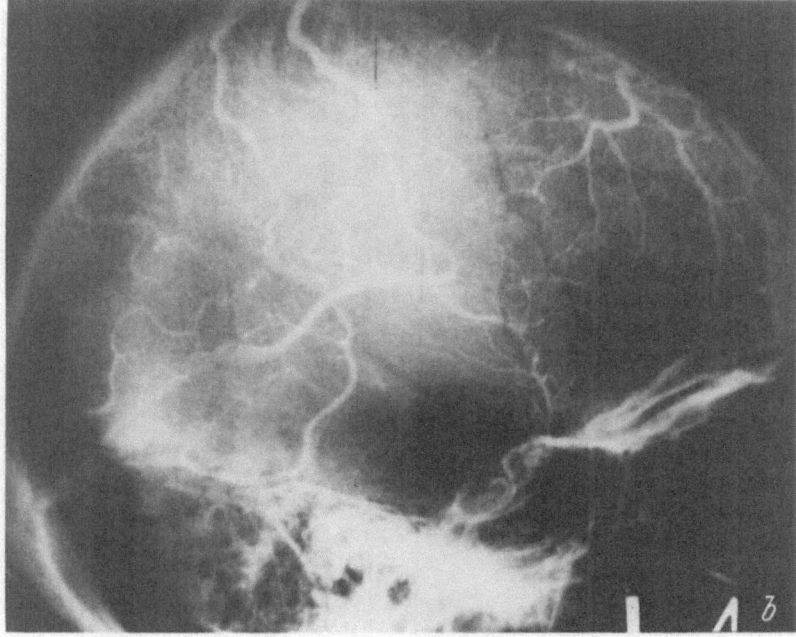

Fig. 15 b

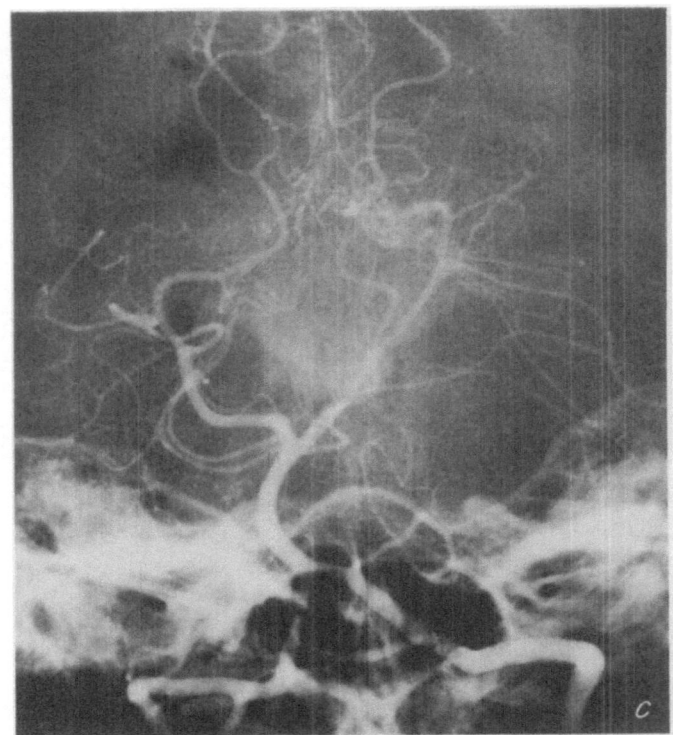

Fig. 15 c

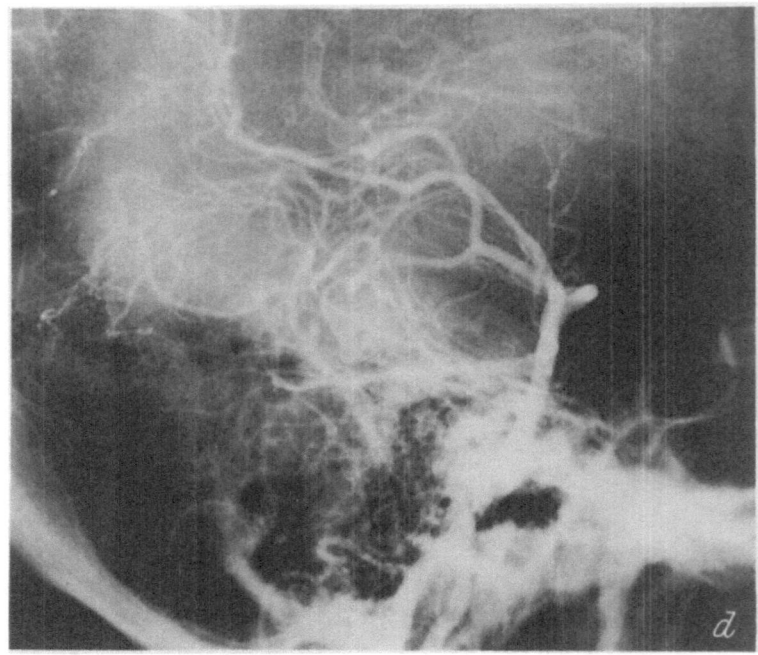

Fig. 15 d

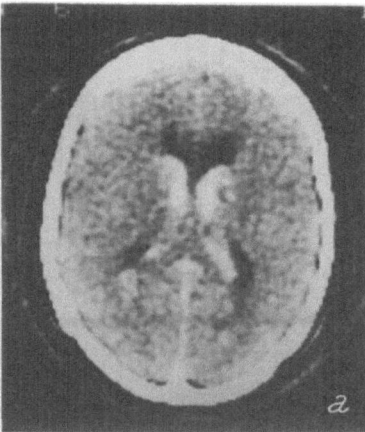

Fig. 16. An arteriovenous malformation on the postero-lateral aspect of the upper brain stem in the region of the superior colliculus. The patient, a lady of 42 had sustained a coma producing subarachnoid haemorrhage, succeeded by confusion and disordered ocular movements. CT scan (a) showed blood in the tela choroidea and a little in the left lateral ventricle. Lateral vertebral arteriography (b) showed the position of the malformation, apparently supplied by the posterior cerebral artery, and draining directly into the vein of Galen. AP carotid arteriography (c) confirmed the supply from the posterior cerebral artery, but at exploration through a combined supra- and infratentorial approach with division of the lateral sinus and tentorium, the malformation was found on the postero-lateral aspect of the superior colliculus, being supplied directly by an enlarged brain stem branch of the posterior cerebral. The lesion was successfully excised and post-operative arteriograms are shown (d and e). The disordered eye movements progressively settled and now, three years after operation, the patient has no neurological deficit. In such a case, the ease of access provided by division of the tentorium substantially diminishes the necessary retraction of the post-temporal region and aids access to one of the more obscure portions of the intracranial space

cholesteatoma, more frequently fairly dense trigeminal loss in the clivus and apical petrous meningiomas.

By the use of this approach, access may be obtained in the supratentorial compartment from the back of the chiasm and the carotid artery, to the dorsum sellae, and in the infratentorial compartment, from the dorsum sellae to the opposite internal auditory meatus, and down to the foramen magnum. The reduction in retractional trauma to the effected temporal lobe is a striking feature of the situation, and compares notably with the deep middle temporal retraction, necessary, for example, in the mid-temporal exposure described by Drake, where the temporal lobe may be frequently extensively bruised and at risk.

Closure

The division of the tentorium and lateral sinus makes a complete dural closure in this procedure virtually impossible. It is the author's practice to close the supratentorial and infratentorial dura as far as possible, leaving the division

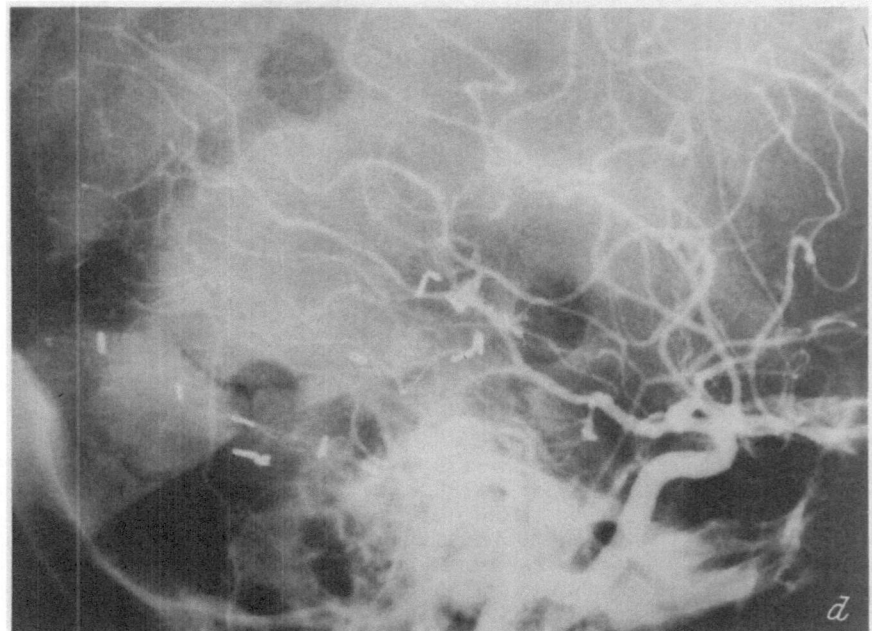

Fig. 16 b

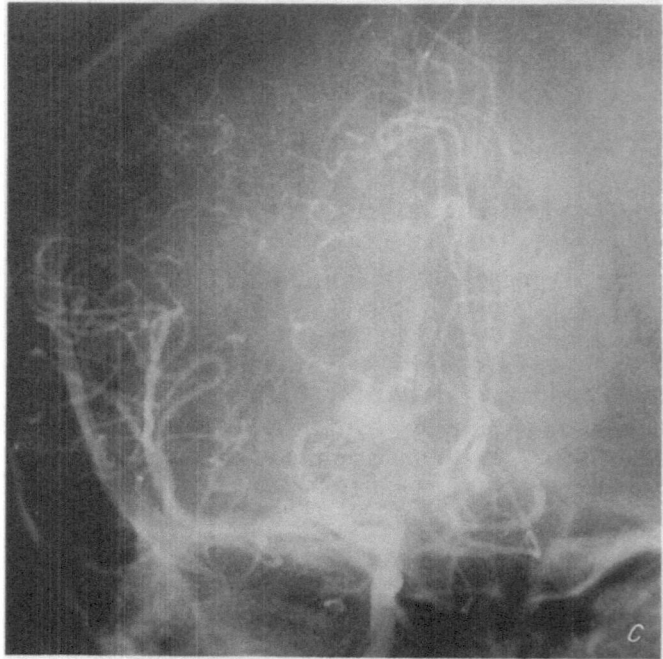

Fig. 16 c

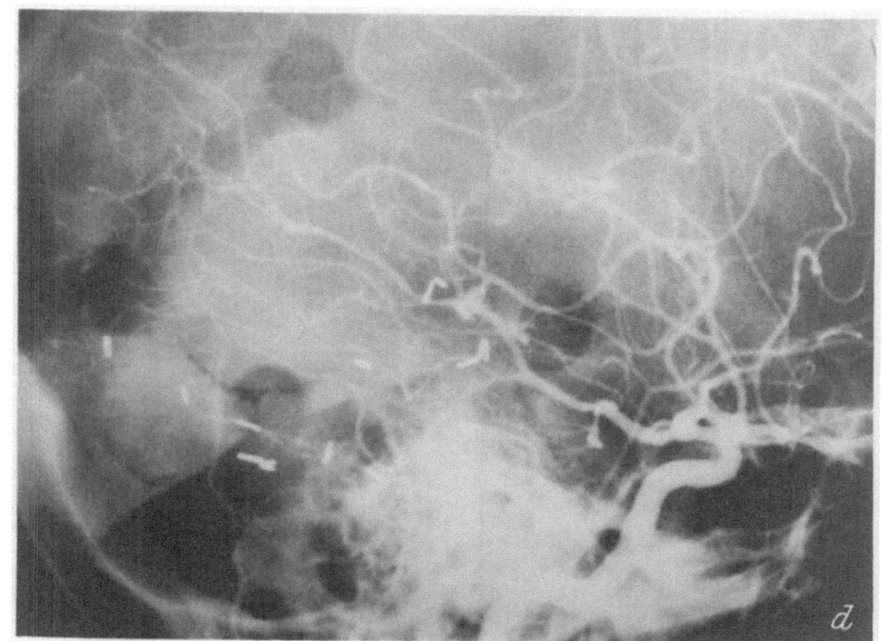

Fig. 16 d

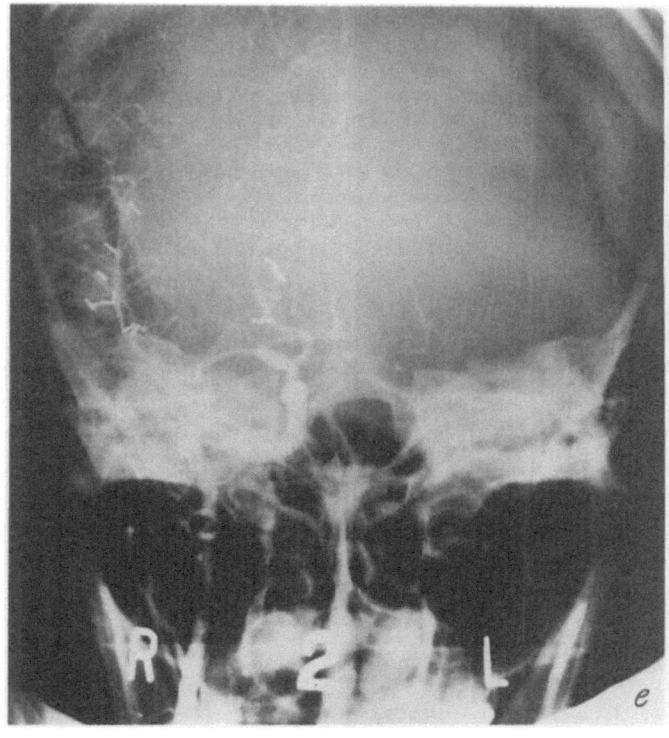

Fig. 16 e

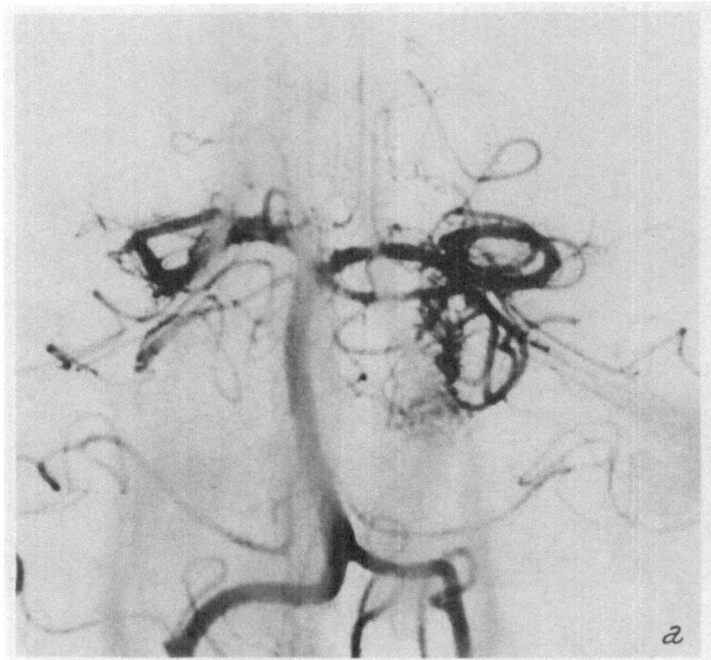

Fig. 17. An arteriovenous malformation in the cleft between the superior vermis, superior medullary velum and medial aspect of the left cerebellar hemisphere. The malformation is shown in the AP subtraction, a vertebral arteriogram (a) and its venous drainage through the lateral mesencephalic venous system, and petrosal vein in the semi-axial sagittal view (b). The lateral film shows the situation of the angioma and the draining vein (c). Post-operative films (d and e) show a complete excision by the combined supra- and infratentorial route with division of the left lateral sinus. The patient had disordered eye movements and upper limb ataxia pre-operatively, and at 48 hours post-operatively minimal word finding difficulties which rapidly cleared. A year post-operatively, there is slight ataxia of the upper limb only, and no other neurological defect

of the tentorium unrepaired, and a defect in the dura over the lateral sinus. This quadrangular defect may be repaired by the insertion of a piece of lyophilised dura (Braun, Melsungen), or of temporal fascia. The other point worthy of emphasis in the repair of this exposure is that in the resection of the petrous base and of the adjacent posterior presenting face of the mastoid, air cells may be opened. The easiest method of dealing with these is to strip off the temporal fascia from the lateral aspect of the supratentorial bone flap, leaving the flap attached only by muscle, and tack down this fairly extended piece of temporal fascia over the base of the petrous bone and posterior part of the mastoid air cells, the fascial flap remaining hinged anteriorly. CSF leaks in this procedure have been uncommon when thus repaired and much less so than in the lateral posterior fossa approach to, for example, acoustic neuromas, where such an extended area of fascia is not available for repair. The supratentorial bone flap is held with a perforating stitch and multiple pericranial sutures, and the posterior

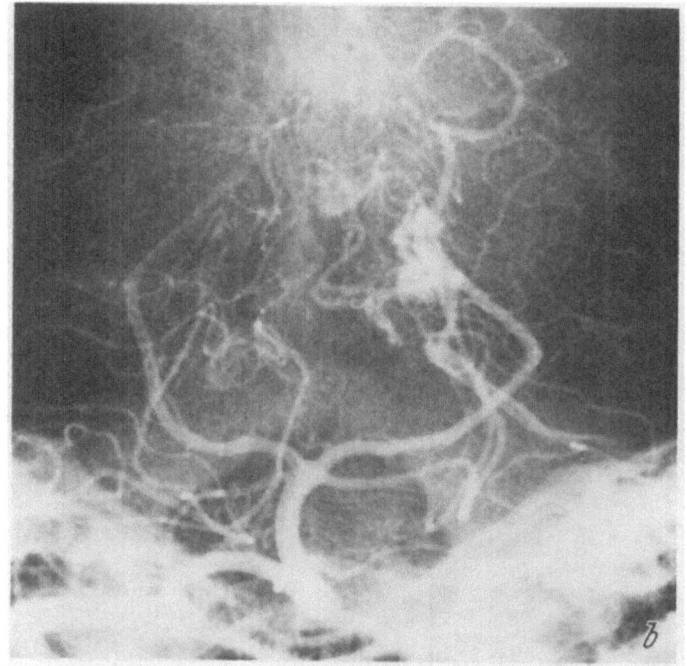

Fig. 17 b

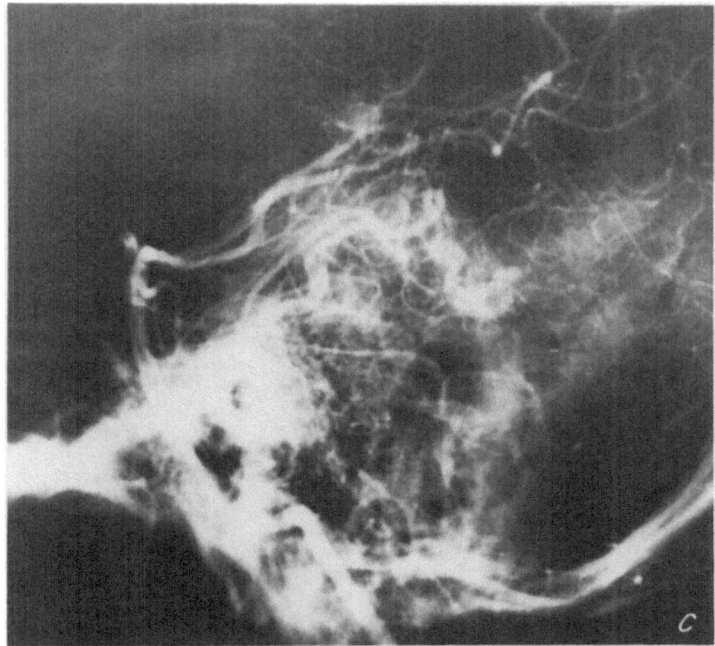

Fig. 17 c

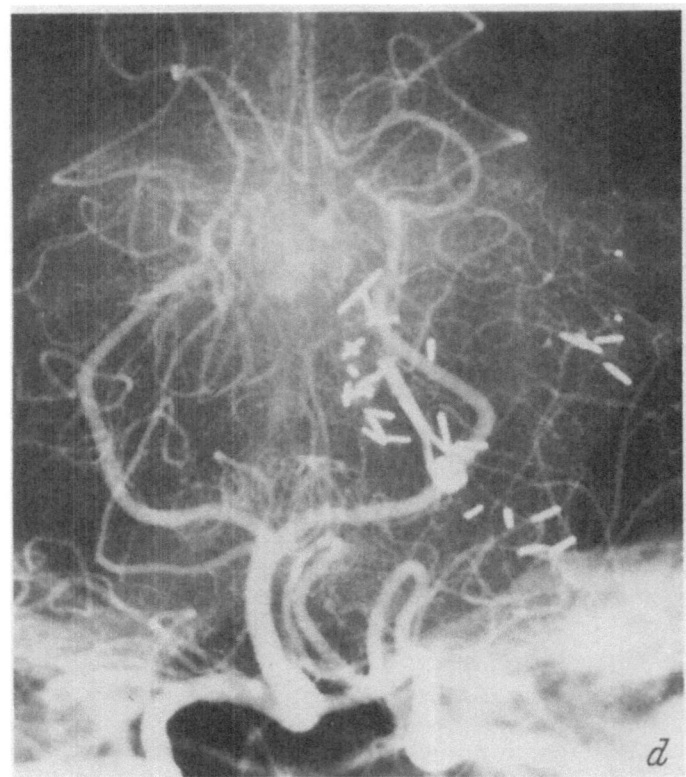

Fig. 17 d

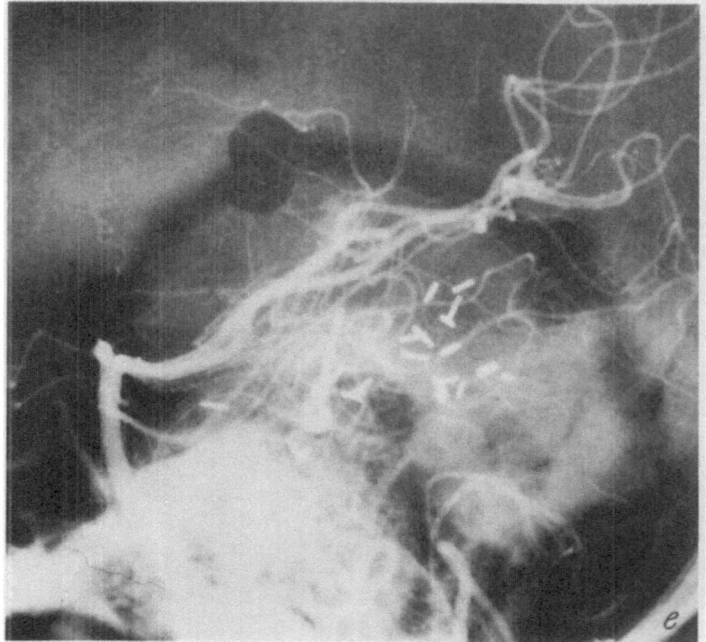

Fig. 17 e

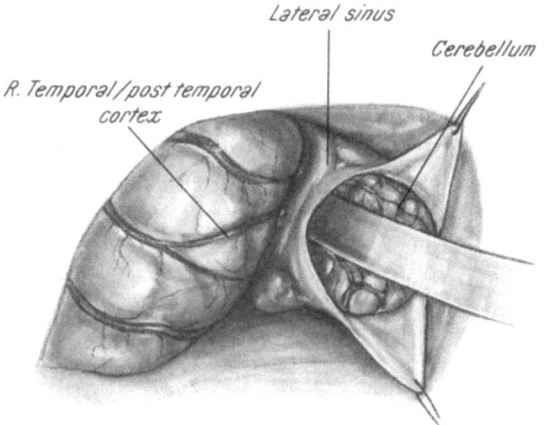

Fig. 18. The combined supra- and infratentorial approach. The supratentorial compartment is exposed, the infratentorial compartment is opened and the cerebellum is being retracted prior to division of the lateral sinus

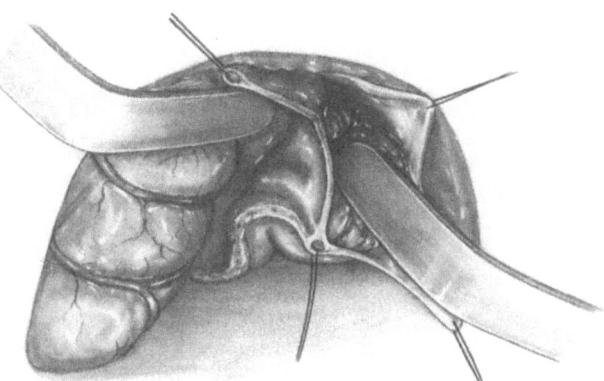

Fig. 19. Combined supratentorial and infratentorial approach, the lateral sinus has been divided and retracted, and the tentorium has now been divided towards the hiatus, the cerebellum being retracted downwards and the posttemporal region retracted upwards

fossa musculature repaired in multiple layers of white silk. The scalp closure is in routine fashion with two layers of black silk, and because of the extensive fenestration of the dura over the region of the tentorial hiatus, it has been the author's practice to omit suction drainage in such cases. Documented brain swelling secondary to the application of suction drainage in cases with an open dura are few, but the author has had several instances where acute brain swelling has followed the application of suction drainage to, for example, temporal lobe in the resection of hyperostotic meningiomas of the sphenoidal wing involving extensive dural resection, and it appears likely that if any suspicion of embarrassment of venous drainage is present in the lobe, then the added negative pressure provided by a suction drain may encourage the development of brain swelling, and is certainly best omitted.

The Posterior Tentorial Hiatus

There are few aspects of neurological surgery which have not been touched by the routine use of the operating microscope, and the practicable microsurgi-

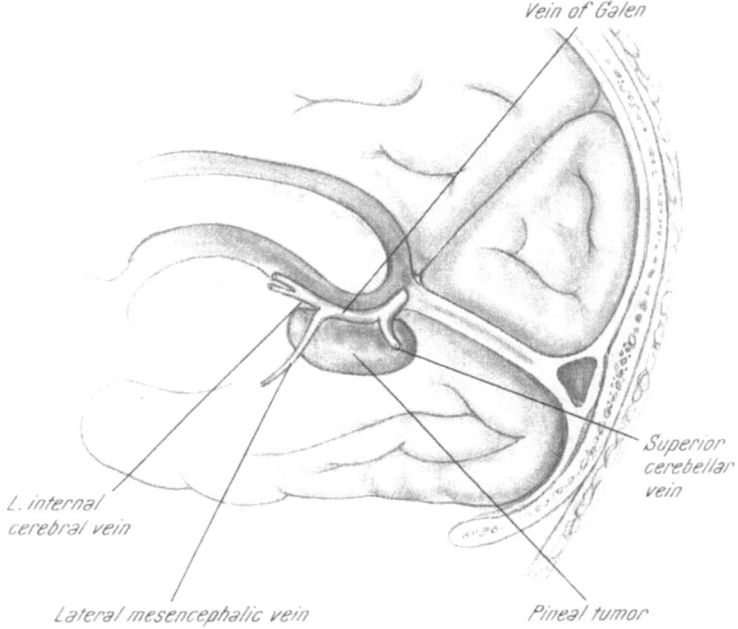

Fig. 20. The situation of a pineal tumour. The approach may be either from above by retraction of the occipital lobe and division of the tentorium, or from below by retraction downwards of the cerebellum

cal excision of pineal tumours represents one of the extensions of the speciality, which may now be regarded as routine. Two principal approaches to the pineal region have been advocated, the subtentorial (Stein 1971, 1977) and supratentorial approach (Poppen and Marino 1968, Jamieson 1971, Lazar and Clark 1974) (Fig. 20). Both are described, the author's preference and routine approach being the latter.

The Occipital Approach to the Posterior Part of the Tentorial Hiatus — the Preferred Approach to the Pineal Region

Positioning the Patient

For this approach, the patient may be either seated or prone. In the author's view, the disadvantages of the sitting position, the risk of air embolism in the close exposure of large venous sinuses, the necessity to retract the occipital lobe against gravity, and the position of the surgeon, who must of necessity work with extended arms, militates against its use. It is the author's practice therefore to adopt the prone position with a good degree of neck flexion and extensive foot down tilt to ensure that the venous pressure is well controlled. The occipital lobe requires scarcely any retraction in the presence of the almost invariable hydrocephalus, which having been drained, allows the lobe to collapse laterally with scarcely any retractor pressure. The surgeon may also operate comfortably with downward directed gaze, not an insignificant consideration as the surgical cervical spine ages.

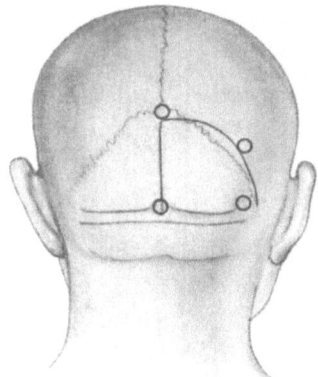

Fig. 21. Situation of a skin incision and a bone flap for the suboccipital transtentorial approach to the tentorial hiatus

The Incision

The scalp incision is a triangular incision which runs from the exion along the midline to just below the parietal convexity, and then turns down to approximately the level of the lateral sinus. The aim of the approach is to cut the bone flap from the midline to the lateral sinus, hinged on the posterior part of the temporal muscle, to enable a clear line of sight along the upper part of the tentorium, and the posterior aspect of the falx (Fig. 21). Once again, the detailed venous angiogram is of particular importance. It is the author's practice to make this approach from the non dominant hemisphere, that is almost always the right side, but the posterior part of the sagittal sinus is sometimes well offset to the right, and an irritating and indivisible shelf of dura containing the posterior part of the sagittal sinus may therefore remain between the surgeon and the midline. In the same way, any extension of the torcular Herophili upwards from the midline, may mean that the ultimate corner between tentorium and falx cannot be completely exposed. These restrictions are usually of little significance, assuming that the ventricular size is adequate to enable drainage to be established early in the procedure, and facilitate retraction of the occipital lobe.

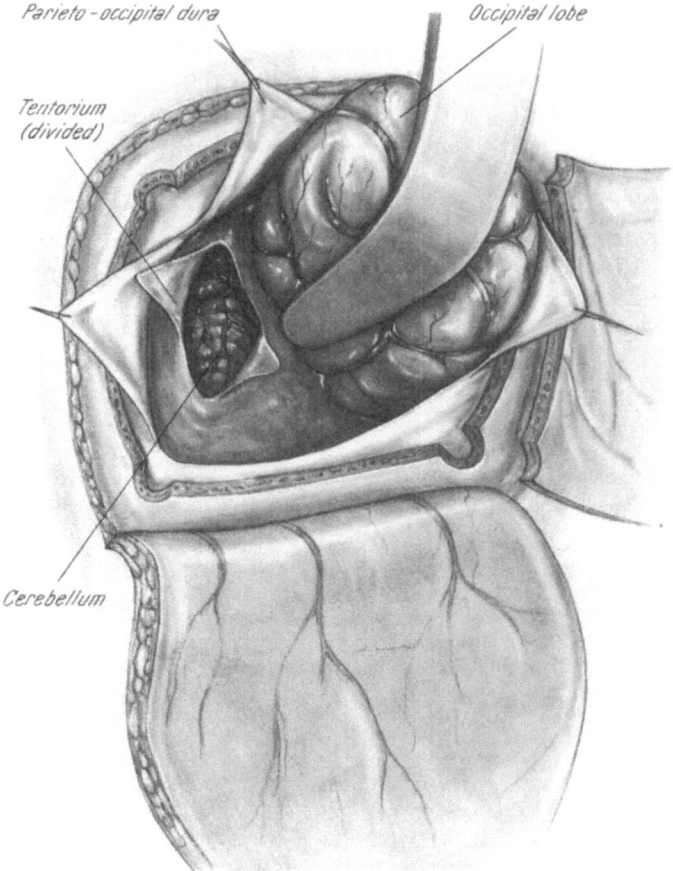

Parieto - occipital dura

Occipital lobe

Tentorium (divided)

Cerebellum

Fig. 22. The occipital transtentorial approach to a pineal tumour, the occipital lobe is retracted laterally, the tentorium is divided and the upper aspect of the cerebellum exposed

The anatomical merit of the approach lies in the virtual absence of veins between the occipital lobe and either the tentorium or the posterior part of the sagittal sinus. It is frequently the case that no veins enter the sagittal sinus behind the post rolandic area, and a segment of several inches of occipital lobe is available in the parasagittal region for retraction without the risk of stretching veins. The dura is opened in a triradiate fashion as illustrated (Fig. 22), the edges held back, and self retaining retraction placed on the occipital lobe, and if necessary, to retract the sagittal sinus and falx to expose the upper portion of the tentorium and the posterior part of the tentorial hiatus. Inspection under the microscope will usually indicate clearly the presence of the straight sinus in the junction of the falx and tentorium, and enable the surgeon to choose a plane of section of the tentorium forward into the hiatus, leaving several millimetres of tentorium

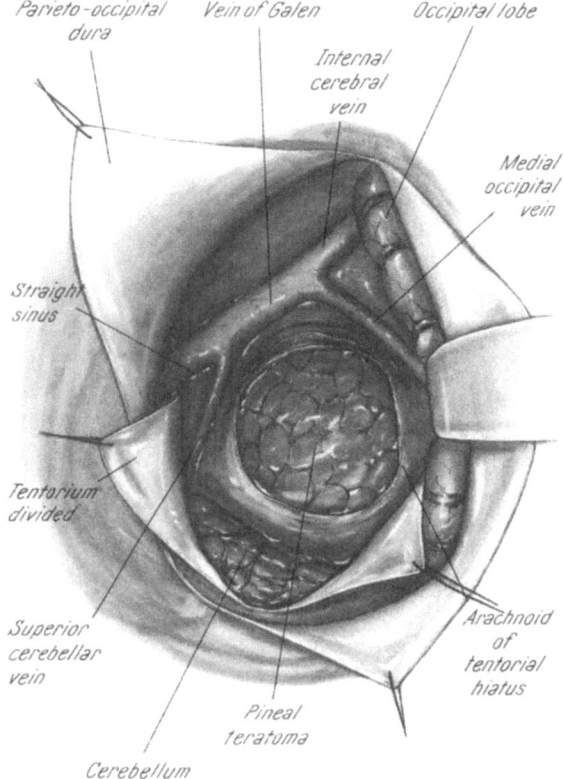

Fig. 23. The occipital transtentorial approach to a pineal tumour, the great vein continuing into the straight sinus is exposed together with the internal cerebral vein and occipital tributary, and a branch from the upper part of the cerebellum. The thick arachnoid over the surface of the pineal tumour had been exposed, the dural edges of the tentorium being reflected. (Drawn from operative video recording)

between the cut and the edge of the straight sinus (Fig. 23). The superior cerebellar veins entering the straight sinus commonly do so within 3–4 millimetres of the midline, and most may be preserved by leaving the cut between 5 millimetres and a centimetre from the midline. The cut should approach the midline as the hiatus is approached, and great care is necessary here to identify the posterior part of the vein of Galen, the veins of Rosenthal, and most particularly, a medial occipital vein which commonly joins the basal vein shortly before it's confluence with the great vein. Injury to this vein is regarded as being responsible for the development of a homonymous hemianopia, which has been the author's only complication in the use of this approach. It should be jealously safeguarded. The arachnoid of the posterior tentorial hiatus is commonly extremely thick, and the pineal tumour, lying as it does substantially below the plane of the vein of Galen and the confluence of Rosenthal's vein and the internal cerebral veins, may not be immediately visible when the hiatus has been opened. Great care is necessary in dissection through this arachnoid to preserve the venous structures of the hiatus and to expose the top of the pineal tumour as it runs forwards into the posterior third ventricle. From this point on however, dissection of the tumour enhances the exposure moment by moment. and the entire third ventricle from the habenular striae forward to the foramen of Monro, is easily accessible by this route. The posterior part of the corpus callosum which forms the upper limit of the exposure has on occasion been divided by other authors, but this has never proved necessary in any personal

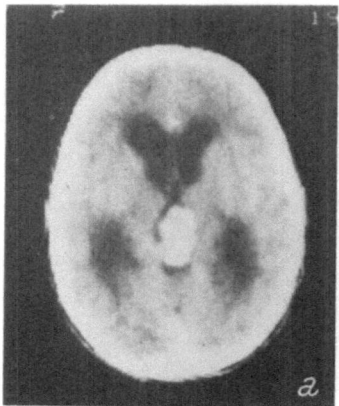 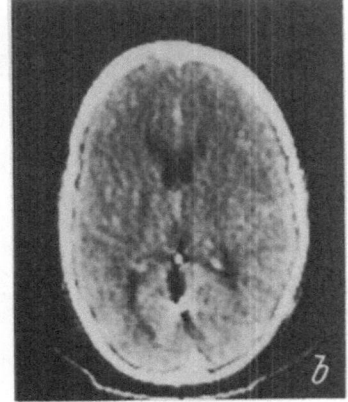

Fig. 24. Pre- and post-operative (a and b) CT scans of the pineal tumour whose operative illustrations are shown in Figs. 22 and 23. The patient, a 12-year-old boy with premature puberty, presented with Parinaud's syndrome and raised intracranial pressure. The tumour, a pineal teratoma, was successfully excised by the supratentorial route. A course of whole neuraxial irradiation was given post-operatively. The boy is well three years after excision

case. Complete removal of pineal tumours of non-invasive type is possible by this route (Isamat 1979). CT scans of a pineal teratoma successfully removed are shown in Fig. 24.

For the rare carrefour meningioma invoving both sides of the falx and the upper and lower aspects of the tentorium, a successive bilateral supratentorial occipital approach may be attempted. These rare tumours however are best approached in carefully staged procedures, the salient problem being the involvement of the straight sinus, quite apart from the frequently enormous size which they reach before diagnosis. The difficulties of the bilateral occipital approach are the hazard to vision, and it may be thought preferable to attempt a limited removal of the contralateral mass through the falx from the original operated side, rather than to attempt to strip a shell of tumour from occipital cortex where vision is retained. The very rarity of these masses makes general statements about the preferred technical approach of little value, and surgery must be planned for each case on its merits.

Closure

Once again the tentorial division is not repaired. If temporary drainage of the lateral ventricle has been employed, it may usually be withdrawn at this stage, it is not the author's practice to leave permanent ventricular drainage in this situation, and the dura is closed with interrupted black silk sutures while the remainder of the craniotomy is closed in the usual way with continuous subgaleal suction drainage.

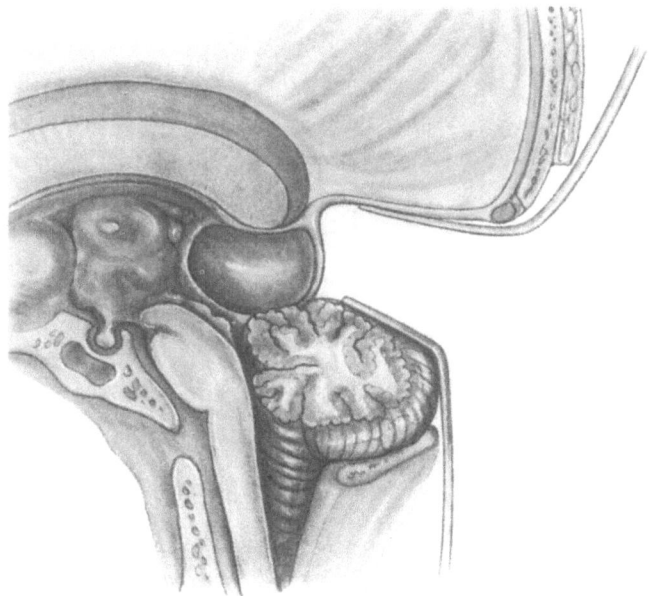

Fig. 25. The subtentorial approach to a pineal tumour. Retraction upwards on the tentorium and downwards beyond the vermis of the cerebellum provides access to the tumour

The Subtentorial Approach to the Tentorial Hiatus

This approach has been primarily used for exposure of tumours in the pineal region, and its chief protagonist has been Stein of the United States. The approach, as he has described it, is best performed in the seated position, after the preliminary establishment of ventricular drainage. An armoured, endotracheal tube, an anti-G suit, central venous (atrial) catheter and positive end expiratory pressure are required to diminish the possibility of serious air embolus, and a further precaution is the use of a doppler apparatus on the precordium. As much flexion as possible should be achieved, since the tentorium slopes steeply upwards, and the line of approach can be quite difficult unless the head is very flexed. A midline or unilateral cerebellar incision may be used, but because of the requirement for extensive decompression high in the posterior fossa, a full cerebellar flap may be preferred. In either instance, exposure of the bone of the posterior fossa must be carried above the level of the torcular, and particularly in the adult, this may involve a good deal of tedious bone work, high in the midline. The posterior fossa bone is exposed from above the torcular to above the arch of the atlas, Zapletal and later Stein have recommended a generous decompression of both cerebellar hemispheres into the foramen magnum including the arch of the atlas. It is best that down to and including the removal of the bone, positive end expiratory pressure be maintained and the G-

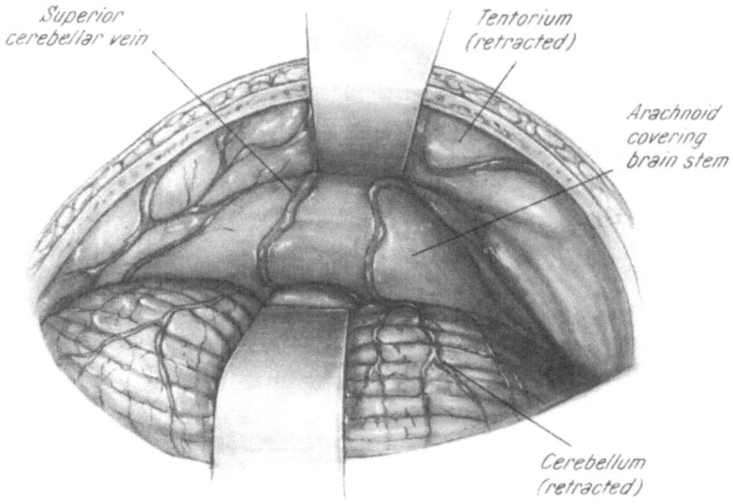

Fig. 26. Stein's (subtentorial) approach to the tentorial hiatus. The vermis of the cerebellum is retracted downwards, the tentorium upwards, and the thick arachnoid overlying the midbrain is visible with draining cerebellar veins running upwards

suit inflated, so that the venous pressure may remain just at the lower level of the wound, and serious air embolus be prevented. When the bone edges have been heavily waxed, and large veins in the region of the foramen magnum, particularly at the lateral angles of Cl have been controlled, then the G-suit may be relaxed, but it is wise to maintain positive end expiratory pressure on the respiratory system throughout. The dura should be opened in a shallow Y, extending from the supero-lateral margins of the craniectomy at the level of the lateral sinuses, downwards and to the midline to divide tha falx cerebelli if present, and the superior edge of this triangular flap held upward with a stay suture while the lower edges are retracted downwards and laterally (Fig. 25). It is then necessary to dissect first in the midline along the superior vermis, dividing the superior cerebellar veins as they pass towards the tentorium on both sides. No harm seems to accrue from the division of these veins, but a relatively long and deep dissection may be necessary to expose the arachnoid of the posterior aspect of the ambient cistern (Fig. 26). Following Stein's advice, it is usually best to proceed from this point onwards under the magnification of the operating microscope, opening the arachnoid of the posterior part of the ambient cistern, and revealing the lower presenting pole of a pineal tumour.

Closure of this approach is not difficult. It has been the author's practice to close the dura firmly, relying on ventricular drainage and steroids to control the post operative swelling, but Stein has advised leaving the dura open, although he admits that troublesome aseptic meningitis may follow, the almost inevitable complication of meningocele consequent upon this manoeuvre.

In Stein's initial report, the cases operated upon were with one exception, (a 14-year-old girl), younger than their teens. Four were between 8 and 11 and one was an 8 month old infant. The smaller the child the more feasible this procedure is. The author has never seen fit to employ it in the late teenage or adult pineal tumours which he encounters, the difficulties of the approach being in themselves not inconsiderable. In the first place, the approach is a very deep one, it requires firm upward retraction of major venous sinuses, and fairly firm downward retraction of the cerebellum, possibly that portion of the brain which reacts least well to prolonged retraction, and it demands the use of the operating microscope in a line of sight which, unless fairly extreme neck flexion can be achieved, points in an upward direction. This position for the use of the operating microscope is uncomfortable, and contrasts notably with the comfortable relaxation of the occipital trans tentorial approach to the same region. Nevertheless, the undoubted satisfaction expressed by notable surgeons in the use of the subtentorial approach, particularly in children, indicates that with practice it may be preferred. The author can only state that where apical subtentorial meningioma in adults has necessitated this approach, it has been difficult and tedious.

Acknowledgements

All the diagrams in this chapter were prepared by Mrs. Angela Christie, in many cases from operative video tape recording. My thanks are due to Miss E. A. S. Wilson for typing the manuscript.

References

Antic, J., Laciga, R., Jain, K. K., Hodosh, R. M., Smethard, E., Yaşargil, M. G., 1976: Microsurgical pterional approach to aneurysms of the basilar bifurcation. Surg. Neurol. 6, 83—91.

Cushing, H., Eisenhardt, L., 1938: Meningiomas—their regional behaviour, life history and surgical end results. Springfield, Ill.: Charles C Thomas.

Davis, L., Martin, J., 1939: Surgical lesions of the paratrigeminal area. J.A.M.A. 113, 1952—1955.

Derome, P. J., Guiot, G., 1979: Surgical approaches to the sphenoidal and clival areas. In: Advances and Technical Standards in Neurosurgery (Krayenbühl, H., et al., eds.), Vol. 6, pp. 102—136. Wien-New York: Springer.

Drake, C. G., 1965: Surgical treatment of ruptured aneurysms in the basilar artery, experience of 14 cases. J. Neurosurg. 23, 457—473.

— 1979: Aneurysms of the posterior circulation. In: Operative Surgery—Neurosurgery (Symon, L., ed.), pp. 263—291. London: Butterworths.

Falconer, M. A., Bailey, I. C., Duchen, L. M., 1968: Surgical treatment of chordoma and chondroma of the skull base. J. Neurosurg. 29, 261—275.

Isamat, F., 1979: Tumours of the posterior part of the third ventricle: Neurosurgical criteria. In: Advances and Technical Standards in Neurosurgery (Krayenbühl, H., *et al.*, eds.). Vol. *6*, pp. 172—184. Wien-New York: Springer.

Jamieson, K. G., 1971: Excision of pineal tumours. J. Neurosurg. *35*, 550—553.

Krayenbühl, H., Yaşargil, M. G., 1975: Cranial chordomas. Prog. Neurol. Surg. *6*, 380—434.

Lazar, M. L., Clark, K., 1974: Direct surgical management of masses in the region of the Vein of Galen. Surg. Neurol. *2*, 17—21.

Love, J. G., Walkman, H. W., 1942: Trigeminal neuralgia and tumours of the gasserian ganglion. Proc. Mayo Clin. *17*, 490—496.

Poppen, A. L., King, A. B., 1952: Chordoma—experience of 13 cases. J. Neurosurg. *9*, 139—163.

Poppen, J. L., Marino, R., Jr., 1968: Pinealomas and tumours of the posterior portion of the third ventricle. J. Neurosurg. *28*, 357—364.

Stein, B. M., 1971: The infratentorial supracerebellar approach to pineal lesions. J. Neursurg. *35*, 197—202.

— 1977: Supracerebellar approach to pineal region neoplasms. In: Current Techniques in Operative Neurosurgery. New York: Grune and Stratton.

Ver Brugghen, A., 1952: Paragasserian tumours. J. Neurosurg. *9*, 451—460.

Zapletal, B., 1956: Ein neuer operativer Zugang zum Gebiet der Incisura tentorii. Zbl. Neurochir. *16*, 64—69.

— 1969: Open mesencephalotomy and thalamotomy for intractable pain. Acta Neurochir., Suppl. XVIII. Wien-New York: Springer.

Management of Chronic Subdural Haematomas and Hygromas

F. LOEW

Neurosurgical Clinic of the Saarland University, Homburg/Saar
(Federal Republic of Germany)

With 6 Figures

Contents

Introduction

Chronic subdural haematomas (Chr. S. H.) have an excellent prognosis if diagnosed and operated upon in time. Because of the straight forward nature of the surgery, the operation of Chr. S. H. is often entrusted to young doctors during their early stage of neurosurgical training as the first operative procedure they are allowed to perform alone within the central nervous system. This article therefore aims to give some guidelines to the young neurosurgeon, what to do and how to do it, to establish an orderly progression of treatments, beginning with the most simple and safe, only going on to more complicated operations if the simple possibilities fail. The reasons of failure and complications are discussed.

Some aspects of the unusual physiopathology of Chr. S. H. have to be outlined, because of the strange fact, different from other intracranial haematomas, that a Chr. S. H. develops only weeks to months after the causative event—trauma, spontaneous bleeding, parainfections effusion. If then tends to enlarge and after mere evacuation without continuous suction drainage, or even after extirpation may have a dangerous tendency to recur.

It is also necessary to discuss briefly some aspects of clinical symptoms and diagnostic procedures before dealing with the proper topic of this contribution, the treatment of Chr. S. Hs.

We have to distinguish, both in regard to aetiology and treatment, between chronic subdural effusions in infants, so-called typical Chr. S. H. mostly of traumatic origin in adults predominantly of advanced age, and chronic subdural fluid accumulations which may appear some time after severe head injury and are found and treated more often since repeated CT scan has become routine in such cases.

Aetiology and Physiopathology

Chr. S. Hs. are caused either by subdural haemorrhage from trauma or other reasons like aneurysm or angioma rupture, coagulopathy etc. or by fibrinous parainfectious effusion. In most cases blood and other fluids within the subdural space are resorbed or organized. Under certain conditions, which are not yet fully clarified, complete resorption does not take place and the organization process, initiating from the inner layer of the dura—intact arachnoidea is not as a rule involved—does not result in the mere fibrosis and dural pigmentation. Instead the cellular elements, which encircle and organize a haematoma, leave some centrally located fluid, which from unknown reasons is not resorbed. As a result the layers of organizational cells on the dural and pial surfaces do not merge into a unified membrane. A fluid filled space results which is surrounded by a capsule of granulation tissue, a neomembrane. This is rich in "giant capillaries", a capillary network of obvious fragility. To explain the secondary increase in size of the fluid filled space, several factors could play a role, as outlined by Weir 1980: increased hydrostatic pressure in the neomembrane's capillaries, increase in its permeability and its surface area, active fluid secretion and at the same time decreased fluid resorptive ability of the neomembrane's cells, or decreased intracranial pressure. In 1932 (Gardner) and 1934 (Zollinger and Gross) suggested a possible increase of osmotic or oncotic pressure in the haematoma fluid. The fact that such pressure gradients never could be verified (Weir 1971 and 1980) cannot be taken, in the author's opinion, as proof of their non-existence. If they do exist, they are likely to result in immediate compensation by fluid movement. In this context, we have to mention also the existence of endothelial fenestrations and open gaps between adjacent endothelial cells in the neocapillary bed, described by Sato and Suzuki 1975. These apparently facilitate fluid movements.

The importance of osmotic/oncotic factors gains in probability from the observations published by Suzuki and Takaku (1970) and others Kurti et al. (1982), who achieved a complete resorption and organization of Chr. S. H. using Mannitol treatment. But this may be followed in old people by increasing of the brain collapse and therefore Mannital may be dangerous.

At all events increase of the haematoma fluid leads to rupture of the fragile capillaries. Accordingly, microhaemorrhages of different age can be found in the haematoma's neomembrane. Such repeated haemorrhages are probably the most important factor which contributes to the progressive enlargement of Chr. S. H. In addition, the haemostatic-fibrinolytic mechanisms are disturbed within the haematoma fluid, as shown by Labadie and Glover 1975, and fibrinogen is absent (Ito *et al.* 1976).

Considering all these factors it is easy to understand that the growth of Chr. S. H. is not a linear process and that even transient reduction in size may occur (for detailed literature see Loew and Kivelitz 1976).

From a historical point of view it has to be mentioned that at first Chr. S. Hs. have been considered as the result of an inflammatory disease of the dura mater, the so-called pachymeningiosis haemorrhagica interna (Virchow 1857), and that a traumatic origin was completely denied. Especially in the German literature Virchow's hypothesis was defended until the late 1960s. Meanwhile it has been demonstrated that the histological picture of the so-called pachymeningiosis haemorrhagica interna is not the cause but the result of subdural haematomas or effusions (for literature see Krayenbühl and Noto 1950, Loew and Kivelitz 1976).

Subdural hygroma sometimes is the result of Chr. S. H. after degradation of all blood and protein compartments and fibrosis of the neo-membrane. In children, especially if it is the result of a parainfectious subdural effusion, Chr. S. H. tends to transform relatively early into a hygroma.

Different from Chr. S. H. are accumulations of CSF like clear fluid within the subdural space which can be found in some cases after severe head injuries. There is no real haematoma, no granulation tissue, and as a rule no capsule. Before the present CT era, this pathology has often been overlooked. The most probable cause of such subdural fluid accumulations is subarachnoid dissection which opens the way from the outer CSF pathways to the subdural space. Only after the initial brain oedema period, when brain atrophy develops and intracranial pressure normalizes, or following decompressive operations, CFS may pass to the subdural space. It seems that in some cases a ball valve like mechanism develops which prevents its backflow. Then a real brain compression result. After evacuation of this CSF collection, the brain expands and its functions improve. In other cases the situation looks more like a brain collapse, and even after external drainage of the subdural fluid for several days the enlarged subdural space tends to obliterate only very slowly. In these cases drainage does not result in impressive improvement of brain function (for literature see Jaeckle and Allen 1979).

Factors Which Promote the Development of Chr. S. H.

Low intracranial pressure, for example following iatrogenic dehydration, CSF hyperdrainagé by an implanted shunt system * (for literature see Faulhauer), or

---

* "If haematoma develops after shunt implantation, the shunt should be closed to facilitate brain expansion, and afterwards replaced or completely removed, according to the clinical picture, to prevent recurrence."

lumbar puncture may cause dilatation of intracranial veins with a possible tendency to spontaneous rupture or at least to more severe bleeding after a traumatic lesion. Bleeding also stops later after accumulation of a larger amount of blood in the subdural space.

A similar situation obtains in cases with cerebral atrophy.

The importance of lowered intracranial pressure with ample space for blood accumulation is stressed also by the fact that after really severe head injuries, which invariably lead to raised intracranial pressure during the initial stage, Chr. S. Hs. almost never develope. They are usually the late results of light to moderate impact. Alcoholics are especially at risk in this respect because they intend to have not only accidents and brain atrophy but often coagulopathy in addition.

In the postoperative period, after evacuation of a Chr. S. H., brain atrophy and lowered intracranial pressure are similarly factors which facilitate the reaccumulation of fluid and blood which may result in a recurrence.

It is self evident that *coagulopathy* is a factor which promotes the development of Chr. S. H., though haematomas, developing for example on longterm warfarin treatment, are often very acute.

Finally the *easy skull deformation of young children*, as for instance during birth or after trauma, may facilitate the rupture of a vein passing through the subdural space and also, by relatively easy enlargement of the skull, may give for the accumulation of blood or CSF in the subdural space.

Clinical Symptoms

Symptoms only start when the enlargement of a Chr. S. H. reaches a degree which surpasses the intracranial space reserve and causes local and general increase of intracranial pressure and a shift of brain structures. Therefore as a rule we find a completely or almost completely symptomfree interval after the disappearance of the signs of the initial event—trauma or whatever—and the beginning of the first haematoma signs. This interval ranges as a rule from one to three months. Only exceptionally are intervals of more than 6 months reported, and then reasonable doubt is justified as to the connection between the haematoma and the reported event.

Following the symptom-free interval is a phase of uncharacteristic symptoms of cerebral function impairment: headaches which are more frequent and longer lasting, an uneasy feeling, increased tiredness with impairment of concentration and so forth. No reliable statistics about these symptoms are available but if the relatives are asked about them, they will usually attest to some symptoms of performance reduction and personality change preceeding the more alarming signs which precipitated treatment.

To enumerate all neurological signs resulting from Chr. S. H. and give a statistical breakdown is of little significance. Sufficient to state that about 75% of all patients present unilateral neurological signs a symptoms, which may even occur on the same side as the haematoma and that psychic disorders are only exceptionally absent. Fluctuating psychic and physical disorders as well as homolateral neurological symptoms are related to the presence of a midbrain cone. One quite frequently sees a varying level of consciousness with the development and resolution of physical signs over hours. In elderly people dementia and ataxia are quite frequent. In bilateral haematomas psychic symptoms are prominent and neurological deficits often absent. As a whole the symptoms are quite nonspecific and therefore, before the era of relatively easy neuroradiological diagnosis, were often misinterpreted.

Chr. S. Hs. in children, newborn and infants display several peculiarities. The clinical picture often resembles hydrocephalus with characteristic fontanelle bulging and head enlargement. If caused by para-infectious effusion, general maldevelopment, irritability and the occurrence of epileptic fits outweigh all other symptoms and can precede the alarming increase in cranial diameter.

Even if the haematoma has been caused by bleeding into the subdural space, its content becomes clear more quickly than in adults. Not infrequently yellow fluid is obtained even at the first puncture as in para-infectious effusions. After further punctures the fluid tends to clear within a relatively short period and to become CSF-like. The haematoma fluid protein level is also lower then in adults and the tendency to secondary haemorrhage is much less. In children bilateral Chr. S. Hs. occur more frequently than in adults and twice as often as unilateral haematomas.

Diagnostic Procedures

In countries where CT scans are available without difficulty, it has become routine almost without thought to get a CT scan in all aetiologically unclear cerebral disorders. Chr. S. Hs. are for the most part, thus diagnosed early enough and all other investigations, which some years ago were necessary to verify the diagnosis, are put aside.

If CT scans are not as easily at hand the diagnostic process should proceed from the less harmful and less expensive procedures to the more complicated and strenous ones. Clinical and neurological investigation, is followed by X-rays of the skull, echography and scintigraphy. Lastly and most importantly, if CT scan is not available, one proceeds to carotid angiography. CT scan and angiographic scintigraphy may unveil an interhemispheric haematoma.

Skull X-rays only exceptionally give proof of a Chr. S. H. if it is calcified, but may help to exclude other intracranial pathologies or, by demonstration of a lateral displacement of a calcified pineal gland, show the side of the space-occupying lesion.

Echography in the form of an A-scan can aid the diagnosis mainly through two findings: demonstration of a lateral displacement of the midline structures and the so-called haematoma echo. Displacement of the midline echo is missing in bilateral haematomas and therefore does not exclude the existence of a Chr. S. H.

Scintigraphy (Fig. 1), nowadays mostly using ^{99m} Tc, gives positive findings both for diagnosis and for localization in about 90% of all Chr. S. Hs. Negative findings have been described in haematomas which in fact were not chronic but subacute and had not yet developed a real capsule, since it is the capsular tissue which concentrates the radioactive tracer.

The characteristic angiographic finding (Fig. 2) is cerebral vessel displacement from the calvarium with the demonstration of an avascular space between brain surface and bone. The shape of this avascular area, the form of the

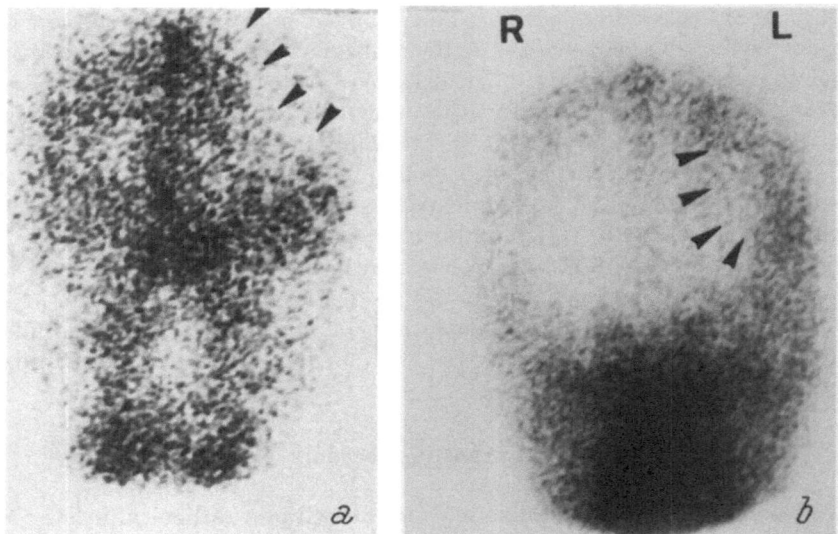

Fig. 1. Scintigraphic findings in Chr. S. Hs. (a) In the arterial phase of a dynamic scintigram the haematoma is characterized by an area of diminished activity. (b) In the static scintigram, which is taken in a late phase, the tracer is accumulated in the capsule of the haematoma

haematoma, depends on its age. A sickle shape is found in acute and subacute subdural haematomas. Planconvex forms can be seen most frequently four to eight weeks after the causative trauma. After an interval of more than 8 weeks most Chr. S. Hs. have a biconvex lens-shaped form. Only in bilateral haematomas does the form remain sickle-shaped or plan-convex (for literature see Loew and Kivelitz 1976).

On CT scans Chr. S. H. may present in at least three different forms: hyperdense, isodense and hypodense (Figs. 3 and 4). All acute haematomas are hyperdense, with an attenuation coefficient higher than the brain. Isodensity prevails in subacute cases but can be found, together with hyperdensity, also in real chronic haematomas. The older the haematomas the more frequent is hypodensity.

Isodense Chr. S. H., particularly if they occur bilaterally, may cause problems in CT diagnosis, but typical compression of the lateral ventricles (Moeller and Ericson 1979) together often with visible displacement of cortical

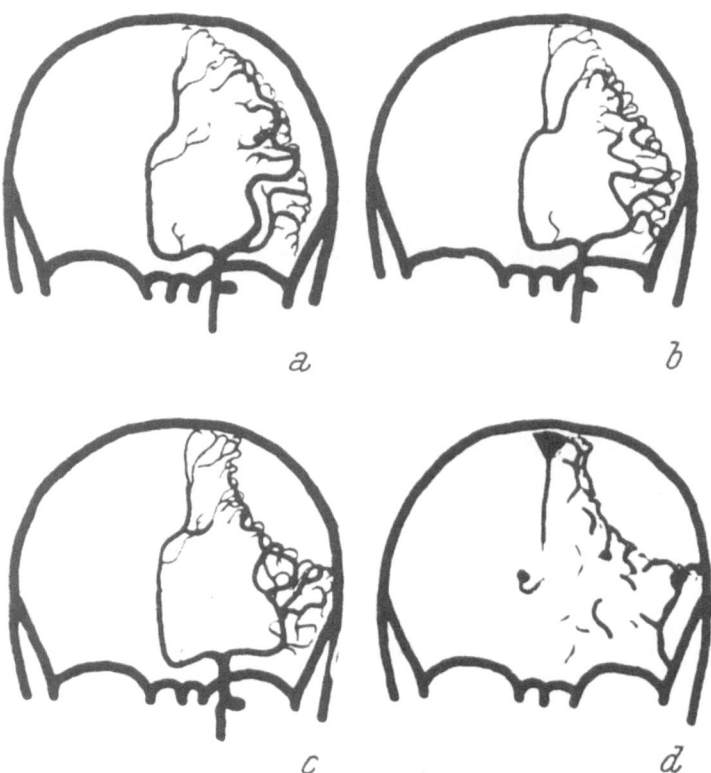

Fig. 2. Angiographic findings in subdural haematomas of different age. (a) In acute and subacute subdural haematomas the cerebral vessels are displaced from the calvarium all over the hemisphere forming a sickle shaped vessel-free space. (b) Plan-convex forms of the vessel-free space are most often to be found between the fourth and eighth week after the trauma. (c) and (d) After an interval of more than 8 weeks most chronic subdural haematomas form a lensshaped vessel-free space (c = arterial and d = venous phase of the angiogram). (From Loew, F., Herrmann, H.-D., 1966)

sulci (Kim *et al.* 1978) and linear areas of contrast enhancement along the medial boundary of the haematoma (Tsai *et al.* 1978) enable a correct diagnosis (for further literature see Markwalder 1981).

Treatment

Conservative Treatment

The "wait-and-see" so-called conservative treatment led to death in almost all cases. Only extremely seldom does the process become inactive or even heals spontaneously (for literature see Bender 1960). If the patients do not die, some cerebral defect is almost inevitable. The rare calcified subdural haematomas are end-results of undiagnosed and therefore untreated Chr. S. H.

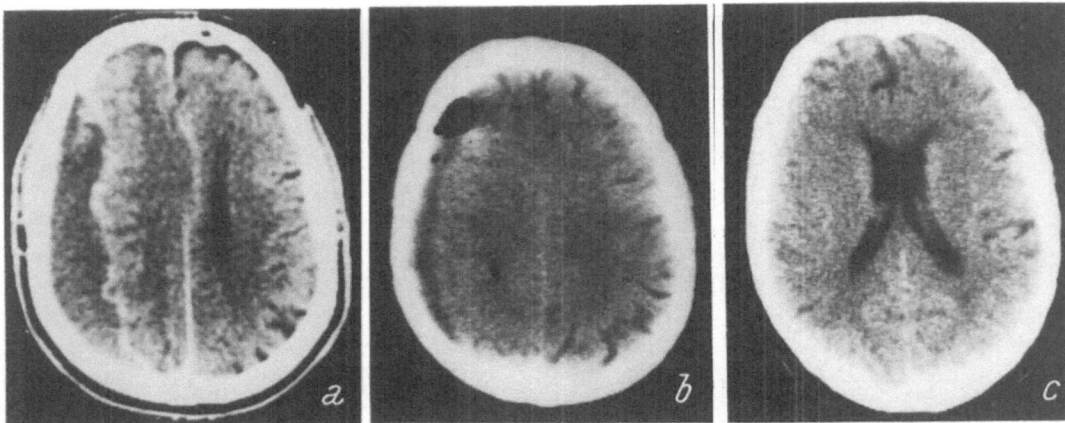

Fig. 3. Example of a hypodense Chr. S. H. Contrast enhancement of the haematoma capsule. The CT follow-up demonstrates also that the resorption of a Chr. S. H. after initial evacuation may take some time. If the patient's condition clinically improves, the doctor should not be worried if a CT control after one to three weeks still demonstrates the existence of a haematoma residuum. In most cases it will be resorbed spontaneously during the next few weeks. (a) Preoperative CT. (b) Even 20 days after evacuation and suction drainage some reminders of air and hypodense fluid are still detectable and the subarachnoid spaces over the left convexity are not yet open. (c) Six weeks later, without special treatment measurements, also the residuum of the Chr. S. H. has been resolved

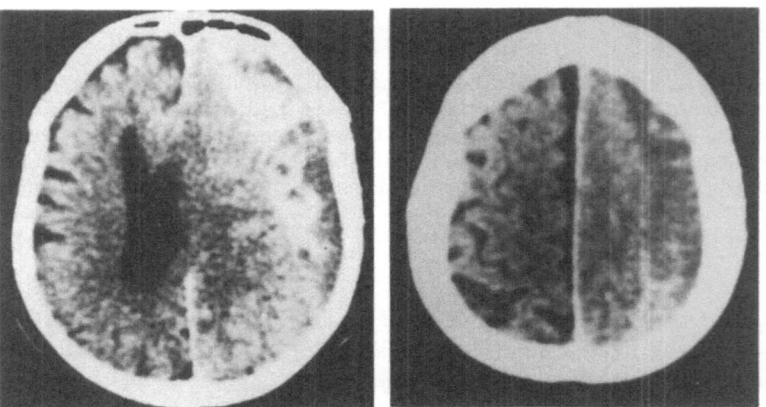

Fig. 4. Example of a Chr. S. H. with CT-hyper- and hypodensities

Real conserative treatment has been initiated by Suzuki and Takaku 1970. They used intravenous infusions of 20% Mannitol, 500–1,000 ml daily with an average total dose of 30,000 ml and an average treatment time of 31 days. In all but one of a series of 23 patients cure could be achieved. Only a few other reports on such conservative treatment have been published (Bender and Cristoff 1974,

Kurti *et al.* 1982), and not all investigators were able to verify similar good results (Gjerris and Schmidt 1974). Since by operative treatment brain compression is released much faster than by Mannitol treatment and therefore brain damage by longer lasting compression can be avoided, since hospital admission time can be shortened and finally that since the results of conservative treatment are uncertain, I would not recommend conservative treatment of any Chr. S. H.

Operative Treatment

The following possibilities to evacuate or extirpate a Chr. S. H. are available:

— fontanelle taps
— burr holes
— external drainage through burr holes or through the open fontanelle
— internal drainage by means of peritoneal or cardiac shunting
— large craniotomy with capsule resection
— reduction of cranial size in cases with extreme disproportion between brain size and enlarged skull size (in children).

Mere evacuation of Chr. S. H. by a single fontanelle tap or burr hole aspiration has a relatively high early recurrence rate. The same is true for large craniotomy with capsule resection, which has to be regarded as major operation and also is complicated by relatively frequent subdural rebleeding and additionally also a risk of extradural haematoma. This is due to the fact that many cases with Chr. S. H. have brain atrophy or lowered intracranial pressure from other causes and that the brain, which has been compressed and shifted over a longer period, does not always expand immediately to fill the place of the previous haematoma. Thus the accumulation of subdural fluid may occur or the development of an extradural haematoma be facilitated.

To overcome these troublesome problems several historical solutions may be mentioned here not as recommendation but to give a more vivid impression of how desperate the situation sometimes can be:

— postoperative lowering of the head of the patients up to 30° below the horizontal for several days
— injection of Ringer solution or air into the CSF spaces by means of lumbar puncture or ventricle tap
— production of cerebral oedema by means of iv-injection of distilled water (Holmes 1953) or cerebral vein clipping (Pia, personal communication).

Clinical experience shows that the resolution of a haematoma can be accelerated and its protein content lowered by administration of a standard Dexamethasone dosage for 4-5 days. This treatment may also be given during 3 to 5 days before operations. Pertuiset *et al.* have insisted on the effect of hormonal therapy.

Nowadays, as a rule, operative treatment starts initially with evacuation of the haematoma by means of burr hole and slow suction drainage for several days or in children with an open fontanelle with repeated fontanelle taps. Only if this fails, are the next steps of operative treatment necessary. In small children the next step should be an internal haematoma-peritoneal shunt. In adults and larger children reopening of the burr hole and fresh insertion of suction drainage or, if from CT examination the suspicion of loculation arises, a second burr hole with subsequent suction drainage over another part of the haematoma helps to achieve capsule obliteration. Only exceptionally a large craniotomy with capsule resection, or even more rarely combined with an operative reduction of skull size, becomes nesessary, manoeuvres now likely to the needed only in very troublesome haematomas in childhood.

Our own material of 261 Chr. S. Hs., 182 older than 10 years (Fig. 5), treated during the last 19 years, demonstrates clearly the policy change which seems to have taken place at the same time almost all over the world. From year to year the relative number of larger trepanations decreased and finally, during the last year, all cases could be cured by burr hole evacuation and suction drainage, or by repeated fontanelle taps. Also the frequency of Chr. S. Hs. in children, resulting from parainfectious subdural effusions, decreased markedly, an observation which probably mirrors the present better treatment of meningitis. Correspondingly also the number of children decreased in whom, by late diagnosis, a very large skull with major discrepancy between brain and skull volume developed. Since 1976 no such child has come to our attention and therefore no operation for skull size reduction has had to be done during the last 5 years.

Technique of Burr Hole Evacuation

Usually this may be done under local anaesthesia. Only in agitated noncooperative cases or children may general anaesthesia be necessary.

The burr hole is placed over the maximum thickness of the haematoma, usually the lower parietal region. A skin incision of about 3-4 cm is made in a coronal direction and the burr hole drilled. A cruciate incision of the dura is made and, if necessary, bipolar coagulation of dura vessels. The haematoma capsule can be opened at the same time or separately. We then introduce a catheter into the haematoma and suck out its brown or yellow content. If some residual clots are present they are sucked out carefully. The haematoma space is then irrigated with Ringer solution. Finally the catheter of a Redon-drainage, the part with its side perforations being removed is placed with its open end into the burr hole so as not to protrude over the inner bone edge into the subdural space, thus avoiding any possible damage to the brain surface if the brain expands. The drain is brought through the skin by a small separate incision several centimeters away from the burr hole, and the burr hole incision is closed by single sutures.

The catheter is connected with a suction pump which allows selection of pressures of 90 or 120 cm H_2O and sucks only intermittently (Gomko Thermotic Drainage Pump, produced by Gomko Surgical Manufacturing Co., Buffalo, N. Y., U.S.A.). Suction is continued about 5 days. The catheter is then removed and a CT scan made. Often some residuum of the haematoma can be detected by CT. If the ventricles have enlarged and the clinical situation of the patient has improved complete resorption can be expected to occur spontaneously. We therefore discharge those patients from hospitalization, but keep them in outpatient control and advise them and the family doctor to come back immediately if any deterioration should occur. It has never done so after the above mentioned management.

If the patients' condition does not improve and CT control shows unchanged haematoma size and ventricular shift and compression, we repeat the suction therapy for some more days. If loculation within the haematoma is visible an additional burr hole over the encapsulated and not yet evacuated part of the haematoma is advisable.

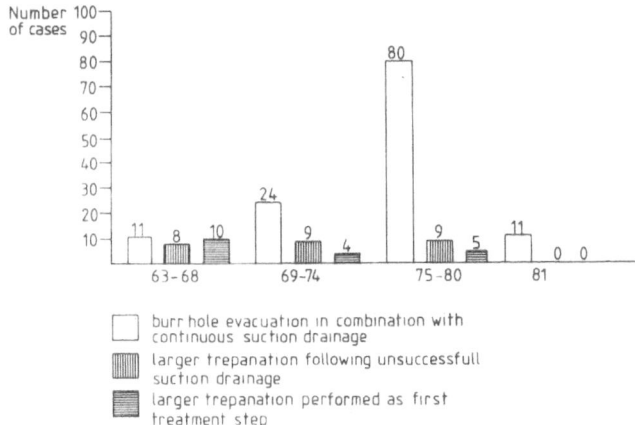

Fig. 5. The figure, which includes only cases older than 10 years, shows clearly that burr hole evacuation in combination with continuous suction drainage has been used more and more as a first treatment and that its failure rate decreased. Finally, in 1981, no larger trepanation had to be done at all

Following this policy, it has been possible to avoid the necessity for larger trepanation and capsule resection in all 11 cases seen in the last year.

It seems advisable to combine the burr hole evacuation and suction treatment with a burst of standard Dexamethasone dosage for 4-5 days. As mentioned before this medication seems to accelerate the haematoma resolution and to lower its protein content.

Peritoneal Drainage of Subdural Hygromas

This operation is indicated as the next stage of treatment in children, when a Chr. S. H. could not be cured through repeated fontanelle taps or evacuation by means of burr hole and suction. As a rule in those children the haematoma has been transformed into a hygroma, and the reason for the failure of the first treatment step is a more or less marked disproportion between skull size and brain volume, due to skull enlargement caused by the haematoma or hygroma.

If this disproportion is not too pronounced shunting of the subdural fluid accumulation will allow readaptation by continued brain growth and by prevention of further skull enlargement.

The earlier hypothesis that the haematoma capsule could hinder brain growth and therefore should be extirpated in any case (Ingraham and Heyl 1939) may be abondoned since Shulman and Ransohoff (1961) as well as Collins (1961, 1965) were able to demonstrate that this is only exceptionally true in rare cases with particularly thick membranes.

Because of complications after cardiac shunts, such as infection of the cardiac catheter and also because the shunt system only has to function for a limited period, peritoneal drainage of Chr. S. Hs. in children, as first described by Collins and Pucci (1961), has become the method of choice. For more recent literature see Njiokiktjien *et al.* 1980. Failures are to be expected in cases with major enlargement of the skull, in which the skull's size has to be reduced operatively (see page 126–128) and in cases with very thick haematoma membranes, in which a larger trepanation with capsule resection (see below) may become necessary.

The technique of haematoma-peritoneal shunting needs no special description, because it is substantially the same as for ventriculo-peritoneal shunts except that the upper catheter is inserted into the hygroma and that many neurosurgeons use an unvalved system with farely wide-bore tubing to prevent its occlusion by the protein rich haematoma fluid.

Haematoma Capsule Resection by Formal Craniotomy (Fig. 6 a–f)

A large skin flap over the maximum haematoma, as a rule the parieto-temporal region, is formed and a bone flap taken out accordingly. The technique of such trepanation is common knowledge and needs no description here. It is advisable to preserve the periosteum and form from it a special flap as large as possible, with its pedicle to the skull base.

The dura mater and the haematoma capsule are opened at the same level. If one dissects the capsule from its dural attachment, multiple small bleeding points become visible on the inner surface of the dura. They may become the source of a recurrence. Therefore most neurosurgeons carefully avoid the separation of any part of the haematoma capsule from the dura. If by any chance the outer lamina had been dissected from the dural flap, we advise removal of this flap and replacement by the periosteal flap mentioned above.

The inner lamina which as a rule has no vascular connections to the underlying arachnoid is resected as far as may be done without difficulty. It should be left in place if it is very attached to the brain. Also its parasagittal parts which often are quite attached to the stretched veins should be left alone.

Normally in the end the outer haematoma membrane is left in place, only the inner membrane removed, the dura closed by running sutures—the running suture has to stop bleeding from the dural edge—with some single sutures in between. In former times the rim of the outer membrane was attached to the dura with clips, but because clips disturbe CT scans, we nowadays avoid their use whenever possible.

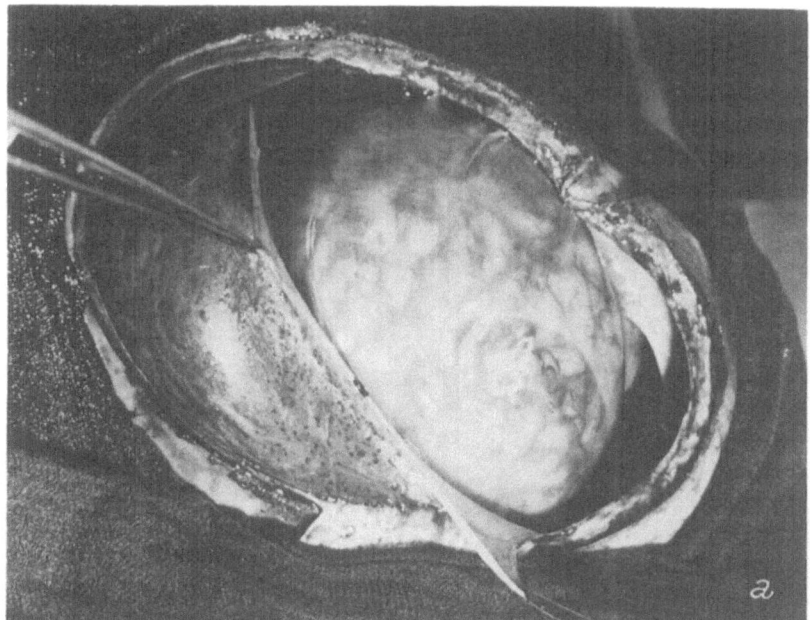

Fig. 6. Operative reduction of skull size. (a) Removal of the outer membrane. (b) Removal of the inner membrane. Note the cranio-cerebral disproportion, the marked thickness of the inner membrane, and the communication to the other side. (c) The dura has been sutured widely on both sides and freed from the "basket handle" like bone bridge. (d) 5-10 cm of the "basket handle" are resected, wire sutures in place. (e) The ends are drawn together. (f) The bone flaps are reduced in size and reinserted

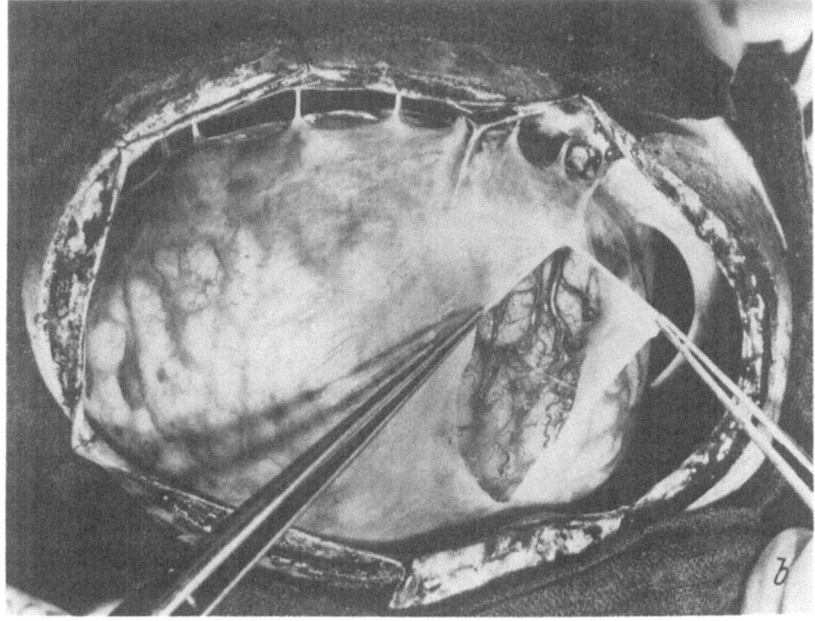

Fig. 6 b

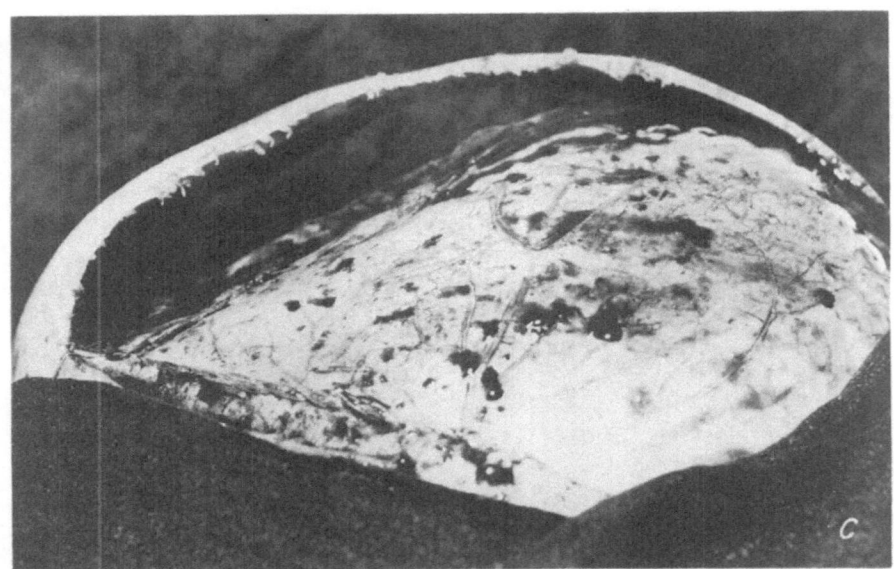

Fig. 6 c

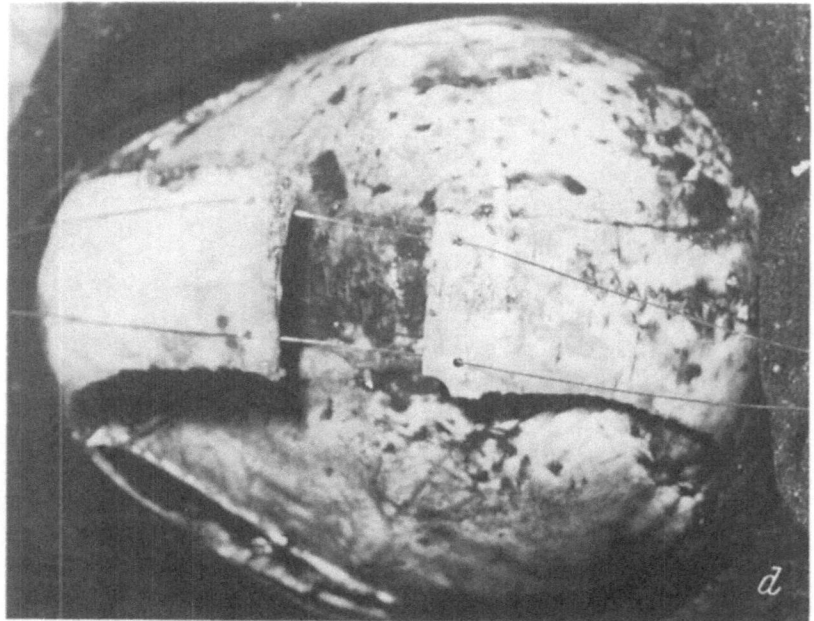

Fig. 6 d

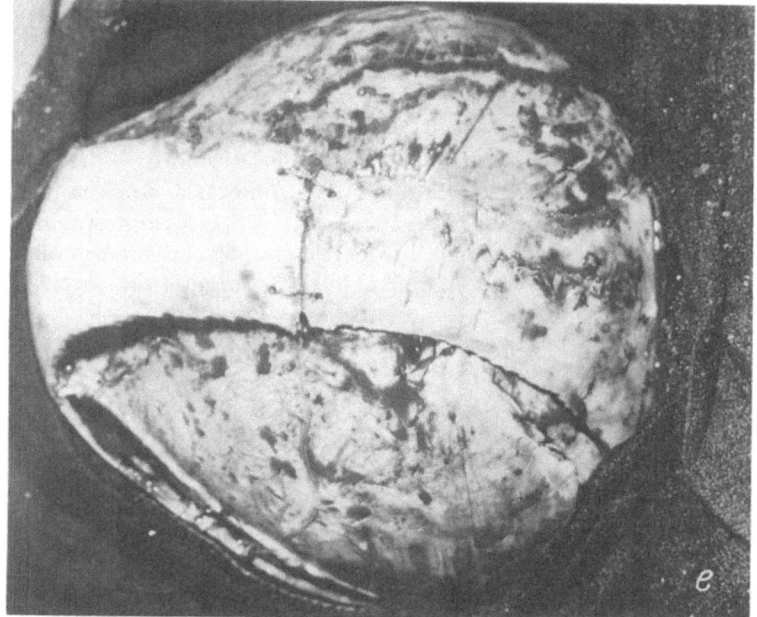

Fig. 6 e

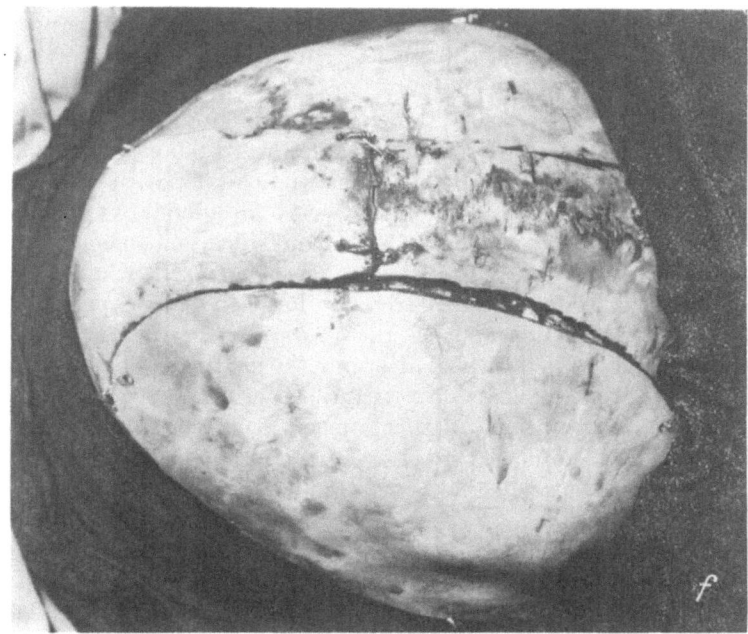

Fig. 6 f

It is advisable to perforate the bone flap with multiple small drill openings of about two millimeters diameter and reinsert it. Using a subgaleal Redon-drainage after closure of the skin, the suction can act through the drill holes. This helps to prevent the formation of a postoperative epidural haematoma.

In some few cases, if in spite of all mentioned precautions either subdural fluid accumulation recurs or an epidural haematoma develops, we remove the bone flap completely, thus allowing the skin to follow the unexpanded and inwardly curved dura. Only weeks to months later we perform a cranioplasty, using the original bone flap as model for an acrylic plate of the same shape as the bone flap, so that it may be indistinguishable from the original, even by the neuroradiologist.

Technique of Operative Reduction of Skull Size

This method, which has been published by us in 1973, is only exceptionally indicated in the now very rare cases of extremely large bilateral chronic effusions in children with marked disproportion between the brain and the enlarged skull (Fig. 5).

After skin incision from ear to ear, large craniotomy and opening of the dura, the outer membrane is excised at the limits of the dural exposure. The removal of the inner membrane is carried out as widely as possible, but care is taken to leave the arachnoid undamaged. If possible the basal cisterns are opened. In the event of marked vascularisation of the capsule, the rim of the outer membrane is attached to the dura with sutures. If the inner surface of the dura bleeds following the stripping of the membrane, the flap is cut off and turned over. Diminuation of the dural space is achieved by suturing the dura closely, so that the dural sac fits tightly to the brain surface. The procedure as described is performed equally on both sides.

The dura is freed from the "basket handle" like sagittal bone bridge, 3-10 cm of the bone are resected and the ends are drawn together with wire sutures. Before reinsertion, the bone flaps are cut down to an adequate fit. Sufficient wound drainage is essential to prevent epidural and subcutaneous haematomas. In most cases the excision of a skin strip is also necessary. The whole operation takes about 2-3 hours. For smaller children the duration of this operation is by no means unimportant. In consequence the anaesthesiologist has to supervise carefully the fluid and acid base balance and the body temperature. In the author's personal series of 19 cases operated upon according this technique, no major operative or postoperative complications occurred, the subdural effusions have been successfully eliminated in all cases, and the cosmetic results were excellent. The head circumferences were reduced as a result of this operation by 3-5 cm.

Long-term follow-up studies were obtained in 16 children. Only five of them, who already preoperatively had severe brain damage with psychomotor retardation, did not improve. The other 11, who had little neurological or mental deficiencies preoperatively, developed into normal infants.

Complications

Acute postoperative haematoma is the most important and dangerous complication. Careful supervision therefore is as important after operative treatment of Chr. S. H. as it is after all other intracranial operations. The incidence in our series was 11 cases out of 182 (6%). Three of 126 (= 2%) occurred after burr hole evacuation and 8 out of 45 (= 18%) after larger trepanation. These figures clearly demonstrate that burr hole evacuation in combination with slow suction drainage is not only the smaller procedure but also far less dangerous than the treatment by larger trepanation and capsule resection. We need not to stress that all postoperative haematomas have to be evacuated operatively as matter of urgency.

Recurrence is different from the above mentioned acute postoperative haematoma. Refilling of the haematoma capsule or, if resected, its former place with a mixture of blood and CSF as a rule progresses only slowly and takes some days to create deterioration of the patient's alertness and neurological symptoms. As shown in figure 4 it can be avoided almost completely by suction drainage and, if it should happen, treated successfully by repetition of the suction drainage. A larger trepanation for treatment of such a recurrence has only been nessessary in 10% of the cases with primary burr hole and suction evacuation and has been avoided completely in the last year's cases.

An unusual and fortunately very rare complication is the postoperative development of a tension pneumocephalus which may delay recovery or even necessitate reopening of the wound (Hirsh 1980, Bouzarth *et al.* 1980). In our material we have seen this complication once.

As after all operations and especially in cases with severe brain function impairment, complications like *wound or shunt system infection, pneumonia, urinary tract infection, embolism* and especially in older patients *cardiac decompensation and infarction* may occur.

Mortality, if not related to special complications, depends on the degree of preoperative disturbance of brain function and of the patient's age. The numbers given in literature reports range from 3 to 13% (for details see Loew and Kivelitz 1976).

In our own material, all conscious patients survived without regard to even very advanced age. Of 37 patients with marked impairment of consciousness or unconsciousness 4 died. They all had an age of 59 years or more. The combination of impairment of consciousness and advanced age results in a poor prognosis.

Results

The late results in children and adults have to be discussed separately, because in children the consequences of Chr. S. H. are often combined with those caused by the lesion which produced the haematoma, *e.g.* meningitis or birth trauma. In both groups they depend to a great extent on early diagnosis and treatment. For literature see Loew *et al.* 1976.

In children about 80% excellent results, that means absence of permanent deficits and normal development, can be expected. In about 20%, mostly due to the underlying disease or damage, cerebral deficit, usually in form of retardation, more rarely as epilepsy and paresis, will last permanently.

In adults good to excellent results have been reported in 80-90%. In our own material 75% became completely symptomfree. 13% had some minor symptoms but were able to do their preoperative work. Only in 12% major disturbances remained. As with mortality, the occurrence and degree of incapacitation correlated clearly to the degree of preoperative disturbance of cerebral function.

Summary

After a short discussion of aetiology and physiopathology of Chr. S. Hs. the main clinical symptoms and diagnostic procedures are summarized.

The methods of treatment available are presented in orderly progression.

The first step is evacuation by means of a burr hole in combination with slow continuous suction drainage, or in young children by repeated fontanelle puncture. In the majority of cases this first step is at the same time the last, and leads to definitive healing.

The second step in children with transformation of the haematoma into a hygroma is an internal hygroma drainage using a peritoneal shunt system. In adults, in which the transformation into a hygroma only rarely occurs, the second step as a rule has to be a larger trepanation with capsule resection.

The last treatment step in children with major head enlargement and marked disproportion of the brain and skull size is an operative reduction of the size of the skull.

Typical complications and results are described.

References

Bender, M. B., Cristoff, N., 1974: Nonsurgical treatment of subdural hematomas. Arch. Neurol. *31*, 73—79.

Bouzarth, W. F., Hash, C. J., Lindermuth, J. R., 1980: Tension pneumocephalus following surgery for subdural hematoma. J. Trauma *20*, 460—463.

Collins, W. F., Pucci, G. L., 1981: Peritoneal drainage of subdural hematomas in infants. J. Pediat. *58*, 482—485.

Faulhauer, K., 1982: The overdrained hydrocephalus. Clinical manifestation and management. In: Advances and Technical Standards in Neurosurgery, Vol. 9 (Krayenbühl, H., *et al.*, eds.). Wien-New York: Springer.

— Herrmann, H.-D., Loew, F., 1973: Operative treatment of extremely large bilateral subdural effusions in infancy. Acta neurochir. (Wien) *28*, 179—187.

Gardner, W. J., 1932: Traumatic subdural hematoma with particular reference to the latent interval. Arch. Neurol. Psychiat. *27*, 847—858.

Gjerris, T., Schmidt, K., 1974: Chronic subdural haematomas. Surgery or mannitol treatment. J. Neurosurg. *40*, 639—642.

Hirsh, L. F., 1980: Intracranial air following subdural hematoma drainage with delayed recovery. Neurochirurgica (Stuttgart) *23*, 55—58.

Holmes, J., 1953: Intracranial hypotension associated with subdural haematoma. Brit. Med. J. *1*, 1363—1366.

Ingraham, F. D., Heyl, H. L., 1939: Subdural hematoma in infancy and childhood. J. Amer. Med. Ass. *112*, 198—204.

Ito, H., Yamamoto, S., Komai, T., Mizukoshi, H., 1976: Role of local hyperfibrinolysis in the etiology of chronic subdural hematoma. J. Neurosurg. *45*, 26—31.

Jaeckle, K. A., Allen, J. H., 1979: Subdural hygroma: Diagnosis with computed tomography. CT: The J. of Computed Tomography *3*, 201—206.

Kim, K. S., Hemmati, M., Weinberg, P. E., 1978: Computed tomography in isodense subdural hematoma. Radiology *128*, 71—74.

Krayenbühl, H., Noto, G. G., 1949: Das intrakranielle subdurale Hämatom. Bern: H. Huber.

Kurti, Xh., Xhumari, A., Petrela, M., 1982: Bilateral chronic subdural haematomas; surgical or non-surgical treatment. Acta neurochir. (Wien) *62*, 87—90.

Labadie, E. L., Glover, D., 1975: Local alterations of hemostatic-fibrinolytic mechanisms in reforming subdural hematomas. Neurology *25*, 669—675.

Loew, F., Wüstner, S., 1960: Diagnose, Behandlung und Prognose der traumatischen Hämatome des Schädelinneren. Acta neurochir. (Wien) Suppl. VIII. Wien: Springer.

— Herrmann, H.-D., 1966: Die Schädel-Hirn-Verletzungen. In: Handbuch der gesamten Unfallheilkunde, Volume 2 (Bürkle de la Camp H., Schwaiger, M., eds.). Stuttgart: Enke.

— Kivelitz, R., 1976: Chronic subdural haematomas. In: Handbook of Clinical Neurology (Vinken, P. J., Bruyn, G. W., eds.). Vol. 24, Part II. Amsterdam-Oxford: North-Holland Publ. Co. and New York: American Elsevier Publ. Co.

Markwalder, T. M., 1981: Chronic subdural hematomas: a review. J. Neurosurg. *54*, 637—645.

Moeller, A., Ericson, K., 1979: Computed tomography of isoattenuating subdural hematomas. Radiology *130*, 149—152.

Nägle, W., 1982: Ergebnisse verschiedener Behandlungsverfahren beim chronischen subduralen Hämatom. Diss. Saarbrücken-Homburg.

Njiokiktjien, C. J., Valk, J., Ponssen, H., 1980: Subdural hygroma: Results of treatment by ventriculo-abdominal shunt. Child's Brain *7*, 285—302.

Pertuiset, B., Chavany, J. A., Weil, B., 1953: A propos d'un coma très singulier — Collapsus cérébral spontané et hématome sous dural secondaire. Presse Méd. *61*, 6, 112—113.

— — — Hagenmüller, D., 1954: Les troubles hormonaux observés au cours de l'évolution d'un hématome sous dural spontané et récidivant. Mschr. Psychiat. Neurol. *128*, 315—326.

Sato, S., Suzuki, J., 1975: Ultrastructural observations of the capsule of chronic subdural hematoma in various clinical stages. J. Neurosurg. *43*, 569—578.

Shulman, K., Ransohoff, J., 1961: Subdural haematoma in children. The fate of children with retained membranes. J. Neurosurg. *18*, 175—181.

Suzuki, J., Takaku, A., 1970: Nonsurgical treatment of chronic subdural hematoma. J. Neurosurg. *33*, 548—553.

Tsai, F. Y., Huprich, J. E., Segall, H. D., Teal, J. S., 1979: The contrast-enhanced CT scan in the diagnosis of isodense subdural haematoma. J. Neurosurg. *50*, 64—69.

Virchow, R., 1857: Das Hämatom der Dura mater. Verh. phys.-med. Ges. Würzburg *7*, 134—142.

Weir, B., 1971: The osmolality of subdural hematoma fluid. J. Neurosurg. *34*, 528—533.

— 1980: Oncotic pressure of subdural fluids. J. Neurosurg. *53*, 512—515.

Zollinger, R., Gross, R. E., 1934: Traumatic subdural hematoma. An explanation of the late onset of pressure symptoms. J. A. M. A. *103*, 245—249.

Subdural Empyema

B. Williams

The Midland Centre for Neurosurgery, Neurology, Smethwick, Warley
(Great Britain)

With 20 Figures

Contents

Subdural empyema (SDE) has always been an uncommon manifestation of intracranial sepsis; when it presents to neurosurgeons in its commonest, spontaneous form it is usually a rapidly advancing disease with a grave outlook. The condition is commonest in the young, and adequate surgery linked to medical care should be capable of producing morbidity free survival; provided that treatment is started sufficiently early and is correctly chosen.

Historical

Macewen described "ulceration of the brain" in his seminal monograph of 1893 discussing all forms of intracranial and intraspinal sepsis. It is this book that provided the starting point of modern systematic understanding of intracranial sepsis and was indeed one of the cornerstones of neurosurgery. Prior to that, operation upon obvious external sepsis, for example those of De La-Peyronie in 1699 and Mursina, Dunville & Watson (quoted by Gurdjian 1969) yielded occasional cures following the release of subdural empyema. Nevertheless before the antibiotic era survival after subdural empyema was a rarity (Kubik and Adams 1943), and when survival did occur it was most probably after craniotomy allowed adequate drainage of a fairly well localised collection.

At the start of the antibiotic era the treatment of intracranial suppuration was revolutionised. Meningitis was no longer a death sentence and the treatment of cerebral abscess was soon altered. Prior to penicillin the preferred treatment was "marsupialization" with insertion of a drain. Macewen used decalcified boiled chicken bones which were absorbable. An account of such treatment given by Jefferson in 1947 who, although welcoming new antibacterial agents, did not recommend tapping and insertion of antibiotics. Nevertheless because of the problems of brain herniation or fungus and the danger of draining early abscesses with thin walls, treatment through burr holes using antibiotic instillation through cannulae quickly became accepted. The application of this principle to subdural empyema followed and the distribution of antibiotics in the subdural space by injection into catheters implanted through multiple burr holes was recommended by Anderson (1947), Schiller, Cairns, and Russell (1948) and Wood (1952). The treatment of subdural empyema and abscess as though they were the same was however, a fundamental misconception. An empyema is, by definition, an infection spreading in a preformed space and drainage by

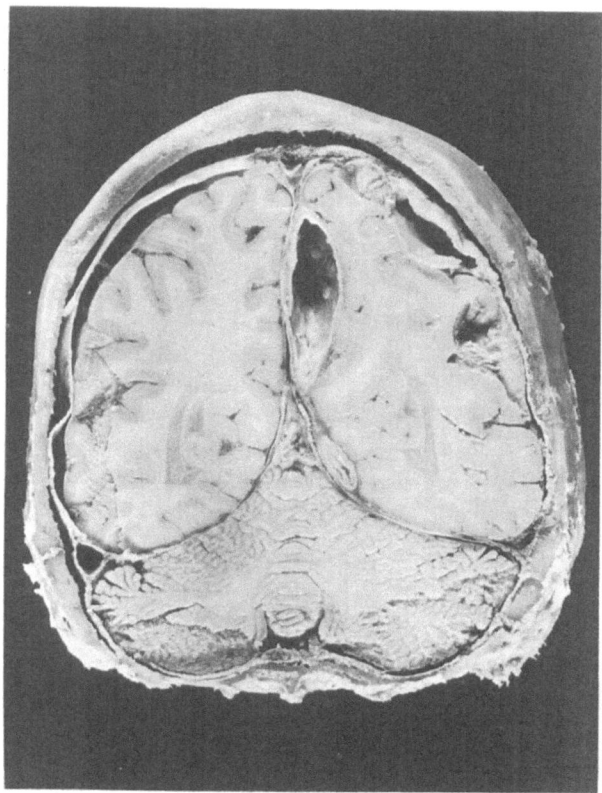

Fig. 1. Post mortem appearances of subdural empyema. Note that the collections are well localised in this instance, the exploratory burr hole just missed a convexity collection in this case. The parafalcine and supratentorial collections are well shown and it can be seen that they would not be accessible to exploration through burr holes. Longitudinal sinus thrombosis is present

insertion of catheters not under direct vision cannot be expected either to provide adequate drainage or to make the instilled antibiotics reach all the living organisms in such a complex space (Fig. 1). The excellent descriptions of Courville (1944) of the preferred route of spread of subdural pus over the convexities, under the frontal lobes, along the sylvian fissure and along the interhemispheric fissure lead to the technique of extensive craniectomy following pus along these situations. The reports of Botterell and Drake (1952) and Stern and Boldrey (1952) showed results greatly superior to these obtained by burr holes. Craniectomy extended to chase after pus above the tentorium is, however, a tedious procedure with subsidiary extensions of scalp incisions and much blood loss. Additionally there is no possibility of a perfect cosmetic result without subsequent cranioplasty. The last case of supratentorial craniectomy was reported by Biehl in 1955. Craniotomy is the preferred treatment, the first sizable series of seven cases coming from Le Beau in 1949. Reports of treatment by burr holes alone continued to appear as late as that of Van Alphen and Dreissen (1976), Joubert and Stephanov (1977) and Van Dellen, Boles, and Van Den Heever (1977).

Bannister, Williams, and Smith (1981) analysed some results from the literature and added 66 cases. They found that craniotomy gave a likelihood of survival around three times better than treatment by burr holes.

Cases in Present Study

The cases used for the bulk of the analyses presented in this paper are patients from the Midland Centre for Neurosurgery and Neurology (MCNN) seen between 1954 and 1981. This series has been reported previously in part (Bhandari and Sarkari 1970, Bannister et al. 1981) and to give a more realistic picture of the disease four cases have been included from the Birmingham Children's Hospital (BCH). This gives 66 survivors and 24 deaths, a total of 90 cases. Unfortunately, some records have been destroyed and some of the tables are necessarily incomplete.

Incidence

Despite improvement in prophyllactic surgery for ear infections, choleste-atomata, and so on, and the availability of new antibiotics, the incidence of subdural empyema does not seem to be decreasing in the middle of England. The Midland Centre for Neurosurgery and Neurology (MCNN) used to serve about $3^1/_2$ million patients. In 1954 this area was served by another neurosurgical unit in the Queen Elizabeth Hospital and also neurosurgeons in the Birmingham Children's Hospital. Since then, two other large neurosurgical units have opened in the Birmingham region and no decrease in the numbers of SDE being referred to MCNN has occurred. In the period 1954-1964 inclusive there were 32 referrals and in the 11 years, including 1971 and 1981, there were 42. Thus we continue to receive about 3-4 patients per year from a population presently served of about 2 million persons (Fig. 2). Infant with meningitis are uncommonly referred to MCNN and of our two infant cases only one could have been due to meningitis although there was scalp sepsis and chickenpox also. This child has not been included in Tables of cause.

Kiser and Kendig (1963) found 8 SDE cases in a series with 129 parenchymatous abscesses (6.2%), Garfield (1969) reported 19% of intracranial abscesses to be subdural. The subdural empyemas constitute about 12% of MCNN referrals for intracranial pus although according to Gurdjian (1969) intracerebral abscess may sometimes be only twice as common as subdural pus. Gurdjian (1969) quoted the incidence of meningitis as being 80 times greater than intracranial abscess (Table 1). Subdural empyema therefore has to be accounted a rarity.

There is a slight sexual bias in our cases of SDE (Males 57, Females 33) although some series have reported a greater frequency of males; the age incidence shows that this is principally a disease of the second decade (Table 2).

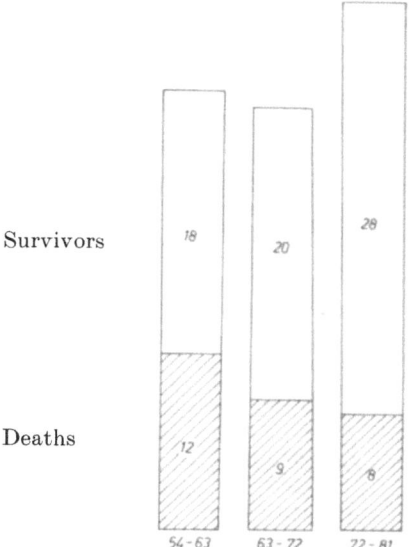

Fig. 2. Histogram of three nine year periods. *i.e.* 1963 and 1972 cases are included twice

Table 1. *Relative Incidence of Intracranial Suppurative Disease*

3,368 Cases (0.6% of 565,253 Hospital Admissions)
After Gurdjian 1969
Mortality in parentheses

	Total	Otitic	Sinus Disease	Overall Mortality
Meningitis	3311 (151)	55 (4)	19 (6)	4.5%
Brain Abscess	39 (7)	5 (1)	6 (3)	17.9%

Etiology

The source of the infection may be a wound or the onset may be spontaneous. The spontaneous varieties are more important because of the severity of the illness and the difficulty in diagnosis. Most of the analyses in this article concern spontaneous SDE, including such causes as spontaneously occuring sepsis elsewhere. Trauma and post-operative causes are not included in the Tables of MCNN/BCH cases except for one due to skull tongs and also cases where instrumentation has been used for surgical treatment of sinusitis. Many published reports however deal with such entities as infection introduced to subdural haematoma by surgery as though they were the same disease as acute spontaneous SDE and discussion may be clouded by this feature. Some articles refer to this class of case as "secondary" SDE.

Traumatic

As a Complication of Surgery

Subdural empyema after craniotomy is well recognised (Wright 1969, Klastersky, Kahan-Coppens, and Brihaye 1979, Reynaudin and Frazee 1980) but uncommonly reported (Coonrod and Dans 1972, Weinman and Samarasinghe 1972, Kaufman, Miller, and Steigbigel 1975, Hitchcock and Andreadis 1964, Post and Modesti 1981). Reluctance to report may be due to a disinclination to confess to complications or because the cases are relatively boring. The organisms are commonly indolent such as staphylococus, serratia marcescens, or diphtheroids. The diagnosis may be relatively easy if a craniotomy site becomes infected. Subdural haematomata form favourable locations for infection after either craniotomy or burr holes (Jacobson and Kane 1954). Infection may be combined with infected valves if the haematomata have occurred after over-shunting. Treatment of these lesions is relatively easy and the prognosis is usually good, no deaths from this complication have been recorded at MCNN.

As a Complication of Trauma

Subdural empyema after other open wounds is again uncommonly reported (McLaurin 1969) and likely to resemble that after elective craniotomy unless the wound has been substantially neglected. Osgood, Dujovny, Holm, and Postic (1975) have reported delayed SDE following injury to the frontal sinus. We have seen one case due to skull traction applied for neck injury, this patient was acutely ill and has not been excluded from the tables. One case reported by Keith (1949) followed impaction of the maxilla.

Spontaneous

As a Complication of Meningitis

Infected subdural effusions are an unusual and interesting complication of meningitis (Hankinson and Amador 1956, Milhorat 1978). Usually seen in infancy and most commonly in patients infected by haemophilus influenza, such collections may be of fluid which is non-purulent or of proteinous or turbid fluid up to frank pus. Clinical signs include failure of pyrexia to resolve, convulsions, head expansion, local transillumination or tightness of the fontanelle with signs of local inflammation (Bell and McCormick 1975). Treatment is dominated by the requirements of the meningitis and the effusions are commonly managed by fontanelle puncture or burr holes although craniotomy may occasionally be necessary. Farmer and Wise (1973) reviewed 17 patients with SDE and in the 8 infants reviewed, 6 had post-meningitic etiology. Four of these infants died with bilateral SDE. No certainly post-meningitic cases have been seen at MCNN.

As a Complication of Paranasal Sinusitis

This is the commonest form of the disease and principally occurs in the second decade of life (Table 2). Sinusitis may have been present for a short while, sometimes even up to some weeks, with localised pain and sometimes eye or scalp swelling. The frontal sinuses are most often at fault although the ethmoids, sphenoidal sinus and even the maxillary antra have been incriminated. Probing or manipulating the frontal sinuses may precipitate contamination of the subdural space (Gurdjian and Webster 1948). One of our cases came on after ethmoid surgery for sinusitis and another after frontal sinus drainage. These are included as paranasal cases in our analyses. Osteomyelitis and/or extradural abscess are likely to co-exist although the combination of subdural and intracerebral abscess seems to be less common. Osteomata and mucocoeles are a significant neurosurgical cause of sinusitis with acute infection (Pool, Potanos,

Table 2. *Age, Survival and Infective Source in 89 Cases of SDE*

	— 10	— 20	— 30	— 40	— 50	— 60	— 80	
Paranasal	2	32	10	5	5	2	2	58
Otogenic	0	7	4	5	3	1	2	22
Miscellaneous*	2	2	2	2	0	0	1	9
Total	4	41	16	12	8	3	5	89
Survivors	3	36	12	4	4	3	4	66

* Includes 3 cases of extracranial osteomyelitis, 3 dental, 1 scalp abscess, 1 lung abscess and 1 cyanotic heart disease. In 1 case the causative lesion was not known.

and Krueger 1962) but no case of subdural empyema due to osteoma has been at the MCNN and in the series reported by Pool no pre-operative intradural spread of infection was noted in 36 cases.

As a Complication of Ear Disease

The second commonest cause in all significant reports except those confined to ear disease, such as that of Beeden, Marsden and Meadows (1969), it is only responsible for one quarter of the cases in the MCNN/BCH series. Otitic disease is more likely to give rise to extradural abscess, meningitis or brain abscess than to subdural empyema. Most extradural abscesses in relation the ear are small and are drained by otological surgeons in the course of mastoidectomy. Of cases referred to a neurosurgical unit with complications of an infected ear, therefore the parenchymatous abscess is the most common. In an analysis of recent MCNN cases Hilton (1981) when considering both acute and chronic ear infection together, found the ratio of intracerebral abscess/cerebellar abscess/subdural empyema to be 7:5:1.

Haematogenous Disease

Many primary sources of presumed haematogenous spread are quoted including 3 dental cases from Hollin, Hayashi, and Gross (1976) and presumed spread from the renal tract (Genest, Bingham, and Hamilton 1963), most of the large series report occasional metastatic cases. Nine metastatic causes are listed as a footnote to Table 2.

Method of Spread

Direct communication between the SDE and an infected sinus or ear can often be found at exploration. When no such communication is seen it is usual to blame the venous system (Macewen 1893, Kalbag and Woolf 1967). At operation, small thrombosed veins are often seen and purulent material may be seen in the subarachnoid space, particularly clustered around the venous lakes and draining veins alongside the longitudinal sinus. Overt thrombosis of large veins is often seen (Fig. 1) and debate may occur as to whether subdural empyema is the cause or the result of the septic thrombosis in such cases. Where there is no continuous thrombosed vein between the infected paranasal sinus or ear and the SDE then infected emboli may have been responsible after moving along the venous system, although it seems likely that pus thus conveyed might more easily find a nidus in the brain parenchyma than the subdural space. Spread from scalp abscess and from organs such as the teeth, tonsils or parotids may also presumably be along the venous system.

Once within the subdural space the purulent material may spread quite rapidly and become widespread. Courville (1944) described the predilection for the Sylvian and interhemispheric fissures and the ease of spread along the base, especially after frontal sinus infection, which may lead to bilateral infections. Over the greater part of the hemispheres the pus may be quite thin and as the disease progresses attempts at membrane formation may successfully loculate the pus into areas which deserve the description of subdural abscess rather than subdural empyema. The case shown in Fig. 1 had reached such a state and the exploratory burr holes had failed to show pus in the subdural space.

Posterior fossa subdural empyema is found most commonly when the cause is otogenic but pus can run between the arachnoid and the dura of the base at the incisura to produce posterior fossa sepsis. Happily the tentorium is so shaped that pus from paranasal disease, which characteristically spreads backwards as though responding to gravity, most commonly finishes up above the tentorium and on one side only. In the interhemispheric fissure or over the surface it is readily accessible to removal. When it is on the top surface of the tentorium (Figs. 1 and 13) removal may be difficult without a sizable craniotomy.

Radiographic investigation by Transmission Computerised Axial Tomography (TCAT scanning) has allowed spread of pus to be observed after burr hole treatment or inadequate craniotomy (Joubert and Stephanov 1977). The characteristic posterior secondary collections may, of course, be seen at the time of presentation (Fig. 3) and two craniotomies can be planned immediately. It is notable that TCAT scans commonly show that the posterior pus is radiolucent whereas anterior pus in the same case may be isodense with brain and sometimes difficult to see even after enhancing the scans with intravenous contrast material. This may be correlated with findings at operation when the thinnest and most fluid pus is most usually that which is found at the back of the head.

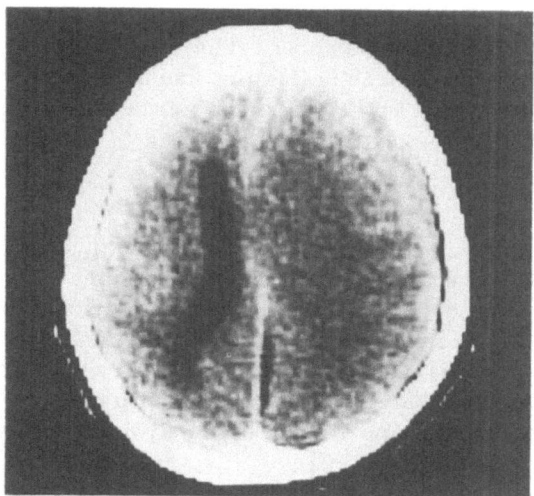

Fig. 3. Characteristic appearance of SDE on TCAT (CT) scans. Same case as Figs. 16 and 17. There is hemispheric oedema, midline shift and obliteration of the ventricle. The subdural collection over the anterior convexity on the right partly enhances and can be seen with difficulty. The radiolucent collection alongside the posterior falx is diagnostic. This case had right frontal sinus opacification on the lower cuts. Hemisphere oedema of this extent invites removal of bone. The parafalx collection demands a second craniotomy (*cf.* Fig. 15)

Presentation

Symptoms had been present for 1–8 weeks before arrival at MCNN or BCH the mean duration being two weeks. The symptoms and signs in decreasing order of frequency (90 cases) were impaired consciousness (68), headache (65), hemiparesis (62), acute fits (55), pyrexia (53), meningism (42), vomiting (27), papilloedema (22), ophthalmoplegia (21), hemianopia (17) and dysphasia (16). It was difficult to grade the patients according to conscious level because many patients had intermittent fits some of which were generalised, and perhaps most importantly the notes have not been kept in a uniform way. Table 4 shows the correlation between conscious level and the outcome as well as the treatment chosen.

The hemiparesis and epilepsy tend to come on together and the paralysis is likely to be total and flaccid from the moment of the first fit. Hemianopia may mean an associated abscess but the usual cause is a collection posteriorly alongside the falx. Such a collection may also give hemisphere signs both motor and sensory, maximal in the opposite leg (List 1950).

Ophthalmoplegia may be due to many causes, local infection in the orbit, cavernous sinus thrombosis and even sphenoidal sinus empyema without intracranial spread may all cause ophthalmoplegia as well as the third nerve and/or brain stem compression familiar to neurosurgeons as a manifestation of the tentorial pressure cone.

Local swelling in relation to osteomyelitis or sinusitis is common as is tenderness over the inside of the upper eyebrow in frontal sinusitis cases.

Perhaps the overwhelming clinical impression in patients with SDE is of the severity of the illness and it's relentless deterioration. It is a condition that once seen is easy to remember.

Diagnosis

The diagnosis in a typical case of subdural empyema is commonly not difficult in a modern neurosurgical unit. Clinical features are usually sufficiently striking to suggest the diagnosis provided that the existence of the condition is known to the clinician. Investigations are usually pursued before craniectomy despite the characteristic clinical features, with a view to arranging the best possible treatment. The chances of the patients also having a parenchymatous abscess for instance are real and a TCAT scan may negate the necessity to probe a swollen brain.

Transmission Computerised Axial Tomography

The history and neurological features usually lead to urgent TCAT (CT) scanning and frequently to immediate diagnosis since features such as extradural abscess, osteomyelitis, opaque sinuses, hemisphere or generalised swelling are all common. The characteristic location of collections of pus is over the convexity and parafalx lucencies are commonly seen usually with peripheral enhancement or enhancement of the adjacent brain. Of the nineteen cases of SDE scanned at MCNN since TCAT (CT) scanners have been in service, fifteen of them came to the department either undiagnosed or with the diagnosis unproven. Only five of these showed subdural pus on the first scan and in two of these the pus was so isodense as to have been misdiagnosed by a radiologist. Most of the scans showed shift due to oedema, osteomyelitis, extradural pus, intracerebral abscess, opacity of the sinuses or any combination of these. Sometimes oedema may be bilateral even when subdural pus is unilateral. An apparently negative result therefore must be regarded with a high degree of suspicion. TCAT scans have given a completely false negative result, *i.e.* a normal scan, in only 1 out of the 15 cases, this was a posterior fossa SDE due to ear disease. The most important observation on the TCAT scan is often the exclusion of a cerebral abscess. In cases in which diagnosis in not clear on the TCAT scan, provided that hydrocephalus and major hemisphere space occupation have been excluded, lumbar puncture will commonly be the next investigation chosen. If the lumbar puncture findings are compatible with SDE then exploratory burr holes made in such a way as to facilitate immediate craniotomy are preferable to awaiting events.

Skull Radiographs and Angiography

In a unit without TCAT scan facilities, straight radiography of skull and sinuses may be helpful but angiography is likely to be diagnostic. The

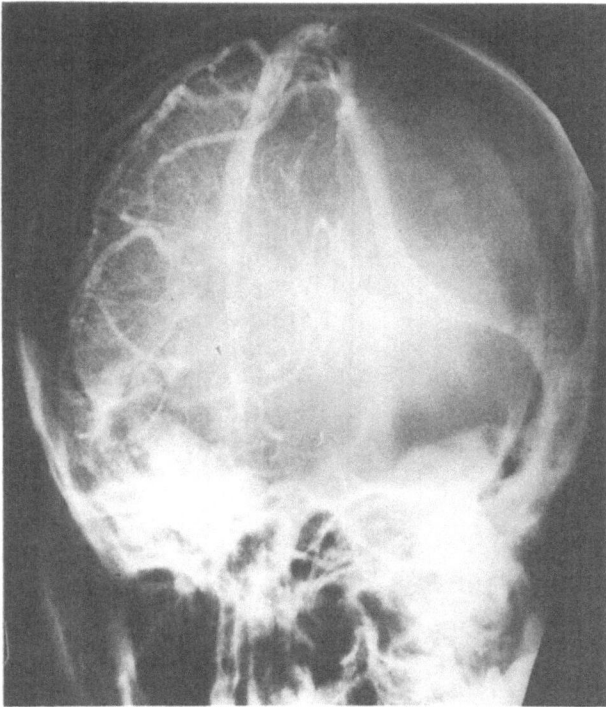

Fig. 4. Convexity collection of pus shown by the gap between the cortical veins and the inside of the skull

Table 3. *Bacteriology of Paranasal and Otogenic SDE (66 Cases)*

	Paranasal		Otogenic		Total	
	Lived	Died	Lived	Died	Lived	Died
Aerobic streptococcus	21	1	3	0	24	1
Anaerobic or microaerophilic streps	12	4	2	2	14	6
Staphylococcus aureus	6	0	0	0	6	0
Bacteroides	2	1	0	1	2	2
Peptococcus	1	1	0	0	1	1
Proprionobacterium	0	1	1	0	1	1
Aerococcus viridans	1	0	0	0		
Staphylococcus albus	1	0	0	0		
Pseudomonas	0	0	0	1		
Pneumococcus	0	0	0	1		
Escherischia coli	0	0	0	1	6	3
Veillonella	0	0	1	0		
Eubacterium	0	0	1	0		
Unidentified	1	0	1	0		
Sterile	3	3	3	3	6	6

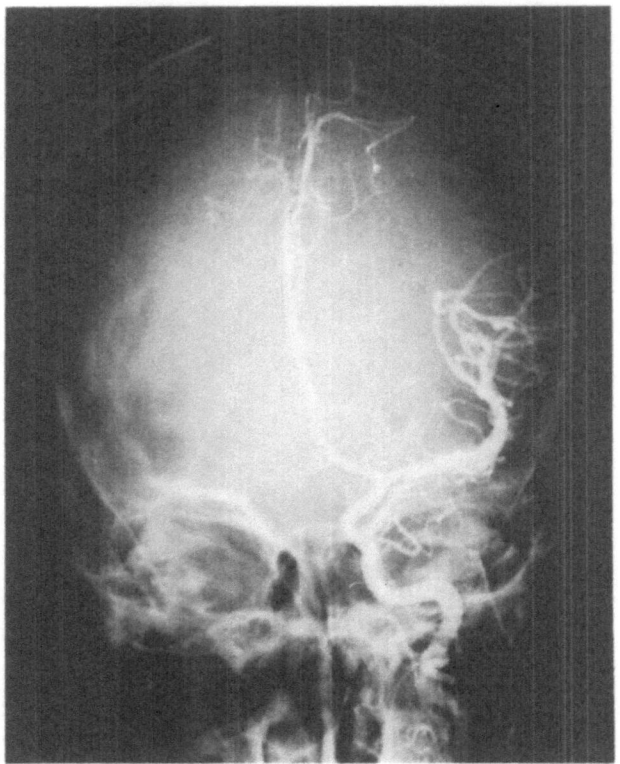

Fig. 5. Angiographic demonstration of the typical parafalx location of pus which demands craniotomy

Table 4. *Treatment Chosen and Outcome in Different Conscious Level Groupings in 45 out of 57 Survivors*

		Numbers		Epilepsy		Hemiparesis		Dysphasia	
		Total	Followed up	Early	Late	Early	Late	Early	Late
Fully Conscious	Burr holes	1	1	0	0	1	1	0	0
	Craniotomy	3	2	2	0	0	0	0	0
Drowsy	Burr holes	7	3	5	1	5	0	2	0
	Craniotomy	18	17	13	6	16	5	4	2
Responding to painful stimuli	Burr holes	9	8	4	3	5	0	2	0
	Craniotomy	9	7	6	3	8	4	1	0
Not responding to pain	Burr holes	4	2	2	1	3	0	1	0
	Craniotomy	6	5	5	1	5	0	1	0
		57	45	37	15	43	10	11	2

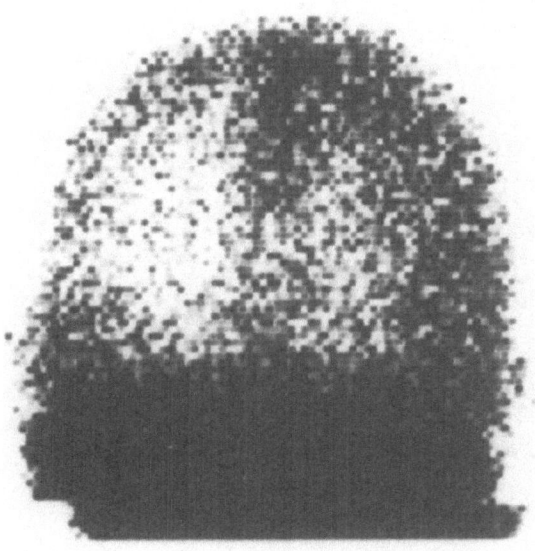

Fig. 6. Rectilinear A. P. scan using Tc 99^m pertechnetate to show convexity pus over the left side and a parafalx collection

characteristic appearances of brain held away from the skull by a subdural collection (Fig. 4) is similar to that seen in subdural haematoma and is often best seen in the venous phase. On the A. P. arterial phase films the interhemispheric collections show as a characteristic bowing of the pericallosal arteries and its branches away from the falx (Fig. 5).

Radio-Nuclide Scanning

In the absence of TCAT scans perhaps the most useful investigation is radio-nuclide scanning (Murphy and Wilkes 1968). In England facilities for rectilinear scanning are more widespread than TCAT scanners. If a computerised tomography of the emission (ECAT) scans are available they help to localise the increased uptake (Figs. 6 and 7). Radio-nuclide scans show osteomyelitis and cerebral abscess well but hydrocephalus, meningitis and encephalitis are not shown and if the diagnosis remains unclear and the patient is clinical unwell then it may be preferable to transfer the patient to a surgical unit with TCAT scanning rather than proceed to further investigation in a unit not so equipped.

Electroencephalography

Widespread disorganisation of the EEG is usual in the typical case. Electrical silence may prevail between fits so that the principal abnormality appears to be in the unaffected side. The diagnosis of encephalitis may be suggested during the early stages of undiagnosed cases.

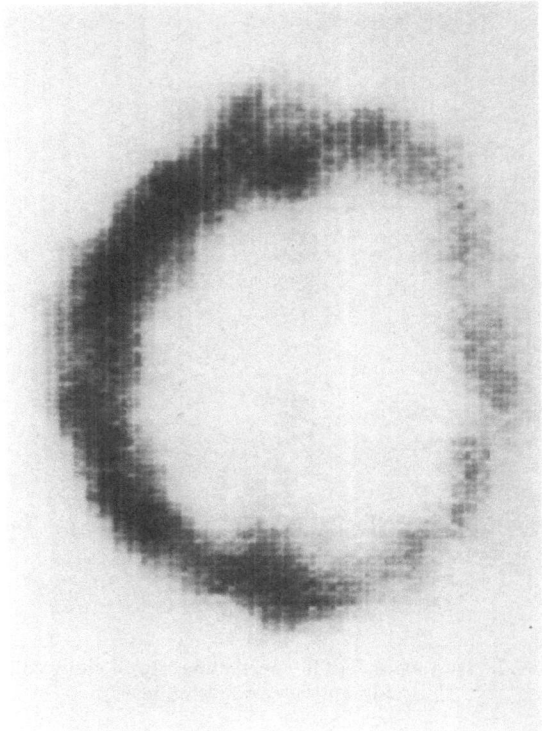

Fig. 7. An ECAT scan of the same case shows the convexity pus well but is a little too low
to show the parafalx collection

Differential Diagnosis

If a patient is admitted with a severe and progressive illness suggesting
subdural or intracerebral abscess the diagnostic possibilities must include
meningitis which may be tuberculous, pyogenic or partly treated meningitis.
The main diagnostic feature of related illness are given in Table 5. Viral
encephalitis is usually due to herpes simplex virus and diagnosis may be difficult
requiring CSF samples separated by an interval of 3 weeks or so to observe
antibody titres rising more rapidly than a marker antibody. Alternatively, a
brain biopsy at craniotomy or subtemporal craniectomy may yield positive
results rapidly by electron microscopy, herpes virus culture or immuno-
fluorescence. Opening the head may also be of help in tuberculous meningitis.
Tubercle bacilli may sometimes be seen on ventricular CSF more readily than on
the lumbar fluid and tuberculosis may also be diagnosable on histology of the
meninges. A caution should be sounded about using immunofluorescent antibody tests for herpes simplex on brain biopsy when tuberculous meningitis is a
possibility, because false positives may result from the use of Freund's adjuvant
containing avian tubercle bacilli (Purdom, Salmon, and Williams 1976). If no

pus is seen in the subdural space in a case without sinusitis, skull osteomyelitis or ear disease it is probably better to await results of ventricular CSF and brain biopsy rather than proceeding to craniotomy. However, if subdural empyema seems a more likely diagnosis than meningitis, or if the brain is very tight and might be helped by decompression, it may be preferable to proceed to craniotomy. Angiography will confirm longitudinal sinus thrombosis which may also be observed at craniotomy.

Table 5. *Differential Diagnosis*

	Head-ache	Hemi-plegia	Convul-sions	Sinu-sitis	WBC's 20,000 +	CSF lymphs over 1,500	CSF sugar normal	Rapid worsen-ing
Purulent meningitis	+	− −	±	−	+ +	Polymorphs	−	+ +
Partly treated meningitis	+	− −	− −	−	+ +	±	−	− −
Herpes encephalitis	+	−	±	− −	− −	+	+ +	±
TB Meningitis	±	+	±	− −	−	±	$1/_2$ *	±
Brain abscess	+ +	+	+	+	±	±	+	±
Extradural abscess	+ +	− −	− −	+ +	+ +	−	+ +	− −
Subdural empyema	+ +	+ +	+ +	+ +	+ +	+	+ +	+ +

* Sugar levels about half normal.
− − Almost never; − rare; ± sometimes; + frequent; + + very common.

Cerebral infarction from an embolus in infective endocarditis may produce a picture much like SDE with an obviously septic illness, hemiparesis, coma and massive brain swelling. A large craniotomy gives such patients a change of survival and excludes localised pus relative to the infarct.

Pre-Operative Management

Airway

If the patient needs to be transferred from a peripheral hospital to a neurosurgical centre the first care should be for the airway. A neurosurgical junior doctor or resident should not be diffident about spelling this out carefully to the referring hospital. Obviously, if the patient is comatose or convulsing then an endotracheal tube will probably be in position, the stomach should have been emptied and an anaesthetist will probably be travelling with the patient. The disasters occur when a patient is put into an ambulance in a fully conscious condition and well able to guard his airway but then develops fits. At the very least such a patient should have a wide-bore stomach tube in position, the stomach empty and intramuscular anti-convulsants given. Sensible precautions for any patient suspected of having intracranial pus include an anaesthetist to travel with the patient taking equipment to intubate and ventilate and a drip in position ready to administer anti-convulsants or mannitol.

Bacteriology and Antibiotics

Ear or nose swabs may have grown an organism which is known to the referring hospital. Subscalp aspiration if there is a swelling may also allow preliminary bacteriology before the patient reaches a neurosurgical unit.

Antibiotic therapy should be started before surgery. Commonly, the patient will have had some antibiotics and the choice of whether to continue or change may be difficult. The range of organisms which may invade the subdural space is very wide (Table 3). Any organism which may cause a cerebral abscess may presumable reach the subdural space. In an analysis of 126 organisms from the most recent 67 intracranial abscesses and subdural empyemas of all types seen in the MCNN, Williams (1982) reported that chloramphenicol was the most successful antibiotic as determined by *in vitro* sensitivities. Of the 126 organisms, 121 (96%) were sensitive to chloramphenicol, 110 (87%) to co-trimoxazole and 100 (79%) to ampicillin. One clear choice therefore is to give chloramphenicol which has excellent penetration of the "blood brain barrier". Because of the slight risk of blood dyscrasias it is rare for this drug to have been given except immediately during the acute illness and we have not encountered any organism from subdural empyema resistant to this drug. A dose of 2-4 G daily for adults parenterally is reasonable and it is usually continued for a week or two in high dosage if the clinical condition and bacteriological findings confirm its usefulness.

It is notable that multiple organisms are less common in SDE than in brain abscess (Williams 1982). The proportion of sterile cultures is high and this is not associated with a good prognosis. Pre-treatment with antibiotics may cause pus to be sterile and also failure to take account of the delicacy of the organisms and the neccessity for cultures to be set up immediately at anytime. At MCNN cultures are begun for aerobic, anaerobic and microaerophilic organisms as soon as pus is recovered from any intracranial abscess; our incidence of sterile cultures has dropped over the years. Yoshikawa, Chow, and Guze (1975) have reviewed the early literature in respect of bacteriology and have stressed the importance of immediate anaerobic cultures and media. Transport media should be arranged if bacteriological facilities are remote from the operating room.

Fits

Systemic anti-convulsants, phenytoin or phenobarbitone can be given parenterally as prophyllaxis but repeated fits sometimes with generalised status justify the use of intravenous diazepam (Valium). A suitable dosage is 50 mgm in 500 ml of saline and administration by a motor driven pump is more reliable than a drip.

The airway should be cared for and in some cases this means paralysing the patients and ventilating for a period. On theoretical grounds the abnormal electrical activity in the brain should be controlled even if the patient is paralysed. A useful review of theory and practical status management has recently come from Delgado-Escueta *et al.* (1982).

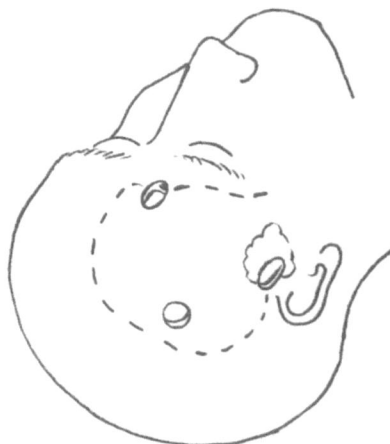

Fig. 8. Suggested layout for exploratory burr holes in an undiagnosed case with suspected right sided SDE. A hole near to the frontal sinus and one close to the ear have the best chance of finding pus. A coronal burr hole over the convexity is convenient for ventricular puncture. Converting the temporal burr hole to a craniectomy allows exploration and cortical biopsy. If SDE is found immediate conversion to craniotomy (dotted line) is recommended

Radiography and Anaesthesia

If the patients are unco-operative and restless, or else convulsing, the TCAT scan pictures are likely to be of poor quality unless the patient is kept still. As with many other neurosurgical emergencies a basal general anaesthetic given before the scan enables the best possible pictures and facilitates straight radiographs, lumbar puncture, or immediate transfer to the operating room depending upon the situation.

Operations

Exposure

Exploratory

If there is a high probability that there is an SDE a bilateral full scalp flap may be chosen within the hair line and this aids in producing a perfect cosmetic result. If the diagnosis is obscure then exploratory burr holes are justifiable with a view to turning them into a flap if necessary. A suggested layout for exploratory burr holes in which right hemisphere involvement might be related to frontal sinus or ear disease is shown in Fig. 8. Burr holes close to the midline are useful to incorporate into a bone flap because if SDE is found, the surgeon must be able to explore the interhemispheric fissure. Additionally, if a bone flap is needed to decompress a tight hemisphere a big flap taken up to the midline is preferable to a small one incorporating a convexity burr hole placed too far laterally. A burr hole low in front of the ear may be turned into a small craniectomy and is useful to allow a temporal lobe biopsy if herpes encephalitis or tuberculous meningitis remain as diagnostic possibilities.

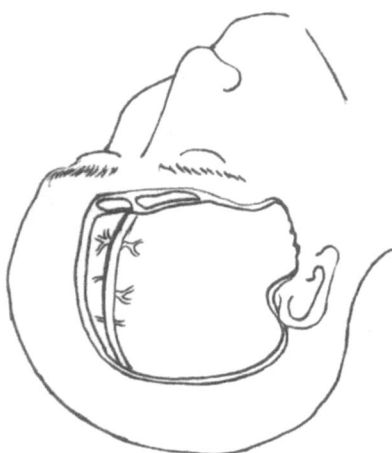

Fig. 9. Suggested exposure for probable right sided SDE due to sinusitis. It is recommended to retain a wide muscular pedicle for the bone flap to maximise the blood supply to replaced bone. A cut low across the sinuses facilitates drainage of one or both of them

Unilateral

If the disease appears to be unilateral and if it seems likely that the bone will be replaceable a large flap can be cut on one side with a wide muscular pedicle left at the base so as to minimise interference with the blood supply. If the flap is taken across the midline (Fig. 9) exploratory nicks may be made in the dura on the opposite side or the opposite side of the interhemispheric fissure may be explored if necessary, although this is uncommonly required. More importantly both frontal sinuses may be explored and drained if necessary.

Bilateral

If it seems that subdural empyemas are probably present on both sides it is probably best to turn two big flaps from the start using the usual transverse flap within the hairline (Figs. 10 and 11).

Posterior fossa

If the disease is well lateralised by either cerebellar signs or unilateral otitis a midline incision with a curve over towards the side of the lesion allows a

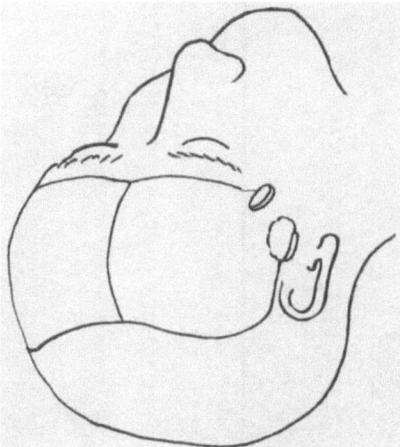

Fig. 10. Suggested layout for a probable bilateral SDE. The flaps should have wide pedicles. If the bone is to be replaced avoidance of burr holes may be helpful in achieving a good cosmetic result but safety demands that the venous sinuses are not damaged

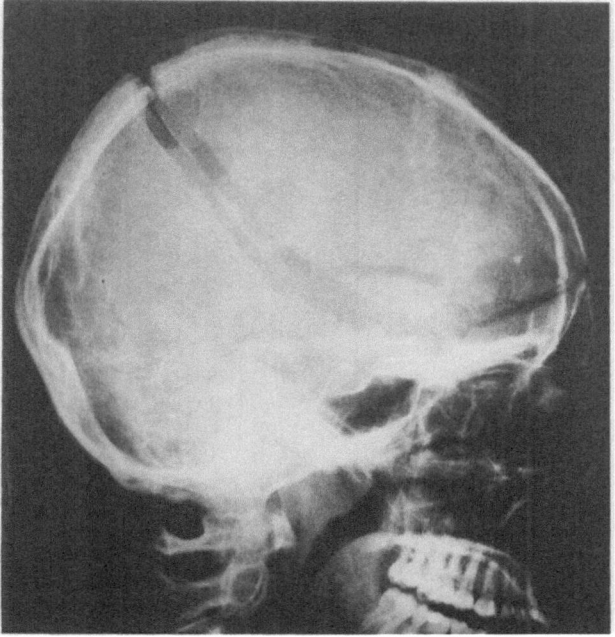

Fig. 11. Bilateral flaps showing perfect healing. This was an otogenic case and the frontal sinuses were not opened

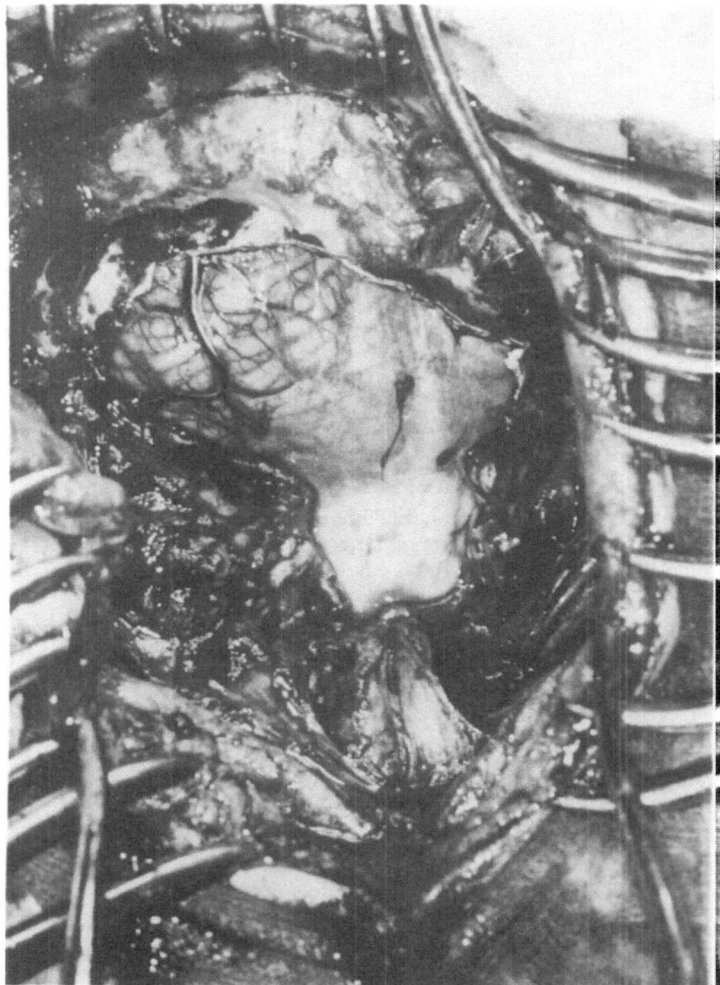

Fig. 12. A left sided posterior fossa craniectomy for SDE arising from the left ear. The arachnoid is intact. Several small collection of pus have been removed and some additional pus is still present on the extreme right. The main collection of pus remained to be released from beneath and in front of the left cerebellar hemisphere. Note that both tonsils are herniated and covered in purulent reactive exudate. The spine of C2 is remaining just below the tonsils

decompression of the whole of the involved side of the posterior fossa. The craniectomy can be taken across the midline and the back of the foramen magnum can be removed to decompress herniated tonsils (Fig. 12). Cerebellar abscess may be difficult to identify on TCAT scans but if the diagnosis remains unclear such approach is helpful in any case of suspected posterior fossa pus; a widespread decompression aids recovery in cerebellar abscess (Griffith 1968).

Dealing with the Empyema

When the dura is opened and pus is revealed the incision should be widely extended to the edges of the wound and the dura may be stitched back. Pus may be localised in one loculus but more commonly there are multiple collections or a widespread layer of pus thicker in some parts than others. The pus may be liquid in parts or solidified in others. Semi-solid pus may be picked off the brain surface with a sucker, washed away and sometimes may be peeled off in strips or plaques. It is uncommonly necessary to use a pattie or pledget of wood to actually wipe it away.

Some authorities have recommended leaving solid materials forming membranes behind (Stern and Boldrey 1952) stating that the inner, cortical surface of the abscess should not be disturbed. Presumably they feared cortical damage. The author's policy is to remove all such material, it is never vascularised in the acute stage and looks as though it may act as foreign material in the maintenance of infection. Clearly in the more chronic stages it may be wise to leave well vascularised adhesions behind.

The arachnoid is usually flattened against the pia with no CSF visible underneath. The surface of the arachnoid may bleed a little and there may be intense hyperaemia of the underlying pia. Ordinarily, capillary bleeding is not a problem. No matter how big the craniotomy the pus is likely to be difficult to remove totally because it is prone to extend beyond the limits. The brain should be pressed away from the inside of the dura using the widest feasible retractor behind the posterior edge. The base of the brain should also be elevated and the interhemispheric fissure should be explored all along its length. If the cranio-tomy is big enough, a site between bridging veins can be chosen to insert retractors and the veins may be left intact. All pus which can be reached should be removed. Exploration of the opposite side is preferable to neglecting a curable collection. When all the visible pus has been removed it is reasonable to irrigate with antibiotics under direct vision at the time of operation. Chloromycetin succinate 1.2 G in saline is the choice of the author, taking care not to leave potentially toxic quantities in pockets where the fluid will not run away. Chloromycetin succinate needs to be broken down to chloramphenicol by esterases such as are present in plasma before chloramphenicol is released. The use of intrathecal chloramphenicol, usually supplied in 2.5 mgm ampoules, might therefore be preferable for quick action either alone or added to the more soluble succinate. The treatment is not intrathecal, it is interthecal and several 2.5 mgm ampoules may be used. It should be used with care when the arachnoid is open so that toxic accumulations are not left behind. Postoperative in-stillation of antibiotics through drains which have been left at operation is sometimes recommended (Stern and Boldrey 1952). Provided that all the pus and avascular membrane is removed however, adequate systemic dosage should produce bactericidal antibiotic levels everywhere within the head (Farmer and Wise 1973). The author prefers to omit foreign bodies such as catheters, and does not instill antibiotics in the wound after operation. The increase in volume of the intracranial contents is undesirable. Catheters may damage friable brain. There is no way of ensuring that the distribution of the injected solution is uniform, it is more likely that the instillation either runs back along the drain or else collects in useless and potentially toxic pockets rather than spreading evenly over the surface of the arachnoid. Hitchcock and Andreadis (1964) comment upon "an increase in seizures during the instillation of penicillin" and opine that "this need not cause anxiety". An alternative view might be that a manoeuvre which provokes fits should cause anxiety since it is reasonable to regard seizures as evidence of malfunction and therefore of toxicity.

The brain may be tightly swollen or may have a remarkably normal volume. In the latter case the dura may be lightly closed with absorbable sutures but in the former case the dura may be left widely open.

If sutures are used then absorbable material is recommended. Foreign bodies should be kept to a minimum although a suction drain is often used to lessen the amount of blood which may remain and provide a culture medium for continued infection.

Care should be taken that the patient does not lie on an area where the bone flap is riding high or else has been removed and it may be wise to build up a dressing around the wound and to write "NO BONE FLAP" on the outside of the bandages.

Second Craniotomies

If the first operation was drainage by burr holes any other response than rapid recovery should lead to a craniotomy. If a craniotomy is small or inadequate (Figs. 13 and 14) a second craniotomy may be required. Secondary craniotomy has been necessary for 24 of our patients as a separate and later procedure. It is sometimes necessary on the opposite side but more frequently the second craniotomy needs to be behind the first. The TCAT scanner is invaluable in observing the postoperative course of subdural empyemas and in a patient where an interhemispheric collection only is seen posteriorly then a small craniotomy at the back to expose the fissure may be helpful. The patient shown in Figs. 3 and 16 had a second craniotomy immediately after the first. Such a flap can be turned through a linear incision a few mm to the diseased side of the midline and after a single burr hole two cuts with a craniotome as shown in Fig. 15 allow an adequate space to retract the hemisphere and to expose the top of the tentorium without damaging the veins crossing to the longitudinal sinus. A small piece of bone like this can be replaced as a free graft. A similar recommendation for craniotomy along the interhemispheric fissure came from McKenzie, (Keith 1949).

Surgery of Associated Lesions

Otitic and Sinus Disease

Some neurosurgeons are prepared to undertake a radical mastoid clearance at the time of operation for intracranial sepsis but for many their training in oto-rhinological surgery is inadequate. Radical mastoidectomy should be carried out early in the illness however, to prevent re-introduction of septic material into the head, and ENT surgeons may also be able to help with such procedures as antral

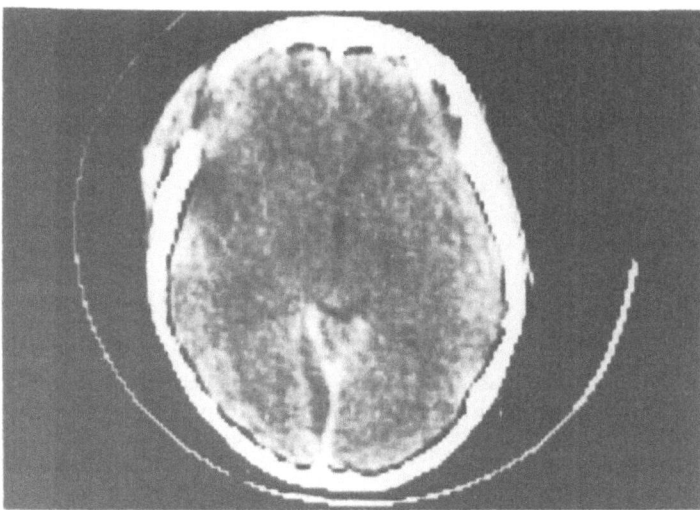

Fig. 13. Result of inadequate craniotomy. The interhemispheric region was not exposed and pus has now run along the falx and collected posteriorly over the top of the tentorium, *cf*. Fig. 1

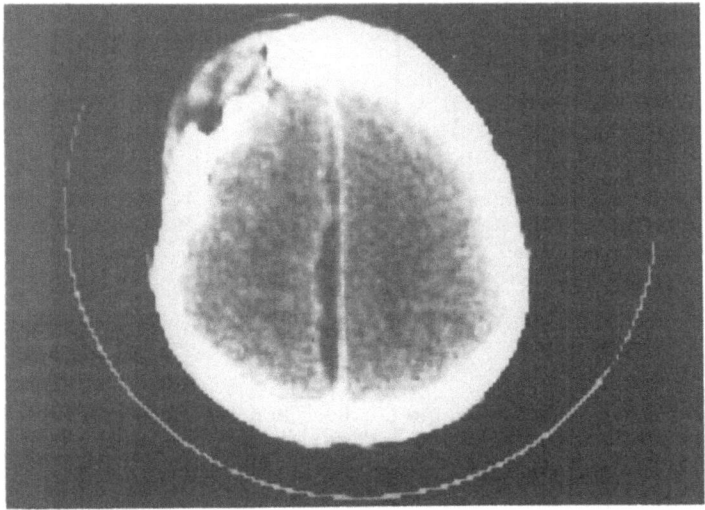

Fig. 14. Same case as Fig. 13 showing the extent of interhemispheric collection after inadequate craniotomy

washouts or transethmoidal drainage of the sphenoid sinus. All neurosurgeons are accustomed to dealing with the frontal sinuses and the method is to take the craniotome or the saw cut low across the top of the affected sinus or both sinuses if necessary (Figs. 9 and 16). The author's practice is to remove the posterior wall of the affected sinus both in the craniotomy flap and also down almost to the

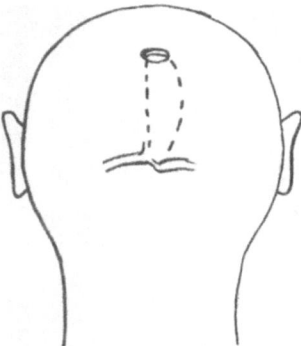

Fig. 15. A small craniotomy based upon a single burr hole may be made through a linear incision. Such a craniotomy allows clearance of interhemispheric collections and exposure of the top of the tentorium

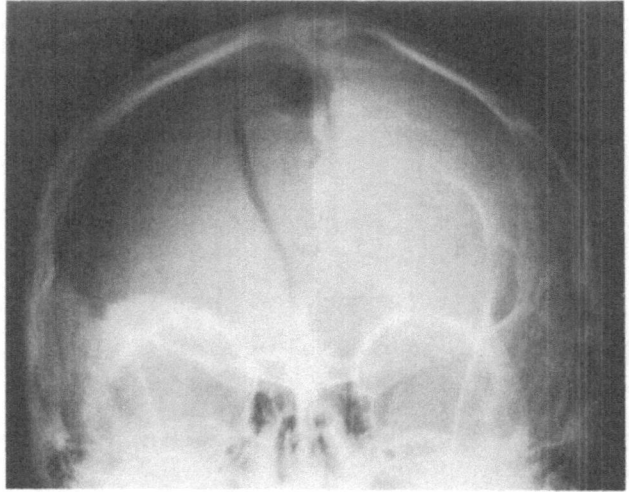

Fig. 16. Same case as Fig. 3. The anterior bone flap cuts across the sinus which was drained. The posterior craniotomy to deal with the interhemispheric collection can be seen, such bone may be replaced immediately as a free graft, *cf.* Fig. 15

cribiform plate and to strip out all the mucous membrane. After identifying the ostium the nose is entered and a drain left from the old sinus cavity down into the nose and out through the nares. Corrugated rubber is suitable. This drain very rarely leaks CSF not only because the surgeon tries not to breach the arachnoid but also because of the massive amount of surrounding inflammation which seals up the openings. If the craniotomy flap is replaced the damaged sinus or sinuses are likely to re-ossify completely. If cranioplasty is required later any residual sinus or attempt at sinus re-formation is usually easily avoided when dissecting open a tissue plane for the insert.

Some authorities such as McLaurin (1969) believe that opening the frontal sinus adds unnecessarily to the time and complexity of the craniotomy and advocate separate and external drainage, the total operating time is however not likely to be much altered and it is reassuring to know that all visible pus has been removed under direct vision at the time of craniotomy.*

Osteomyelitis

Although a small amount of osseous inflammation can recover, if it is extensive, or if there is an obvious sequestrum then it is probably best to take out all the involved bone. If bone is even mildly infected it is best not to leave even absorbable sutures in proximity to it if it is replaced. A posterior free fragment like that shown in Figs. 15 and 16 is obviously partly devitalised and although not previously infected it is at risk. A little fragment like that will however, lie in position without any sutures in the dura, the periosteum or even the galea and the chances of perfect healing are thereby probably improved. If an external cast of all the suspect area was taken beforehand then some of the bone, even eyebrows or bridge of the nose may be removed with confidence that a perfect repair can be done later (Fig. 18). If the part of the eyebrow region comes out as a sequestrum (Figs. 19 and 20) the cranioplasty technician may sometimes be able to reconstruct the fragments and with the aid of wax re-make a perfect prosthesis.

Epidural Abscess

The TCAT scan appearances are commonly clear in extradural abscess, the edges of the collection enhance well and many cross the site of the falx. There is commonly an associated osteomyelitis. An abscess which is entirely extradural is likely to produce no hemiparesis or fits and little in the way of meningism. For such a case therefore if there is no TCAT scan evidence of SDE it is tempting not to open the dura during the operative treatment of a sizable extradural abscess. It may be difficult to see if there is pus under the dura when it is intact. If there is none it is sometimes possible to move fluid easily under the dura by massaging gently with a pattie. If this can be done all over the exposed part of the hemisphere then subdural pus is improbable. If in any doubt however it is probably best to nick the dura and have a look in a few places rather than to send the patient back to the ward with the possibility of further deterioration due to undetected SDE. Obviously the pus from the extradural space should be sucked, washed and wiped away thoroughly before a possibly clean compartment is opened and it is the author's practice to irrigate with a solution of chloromycetin succinate or chloramphenicol before and after opening the dura.

Cranioplasty

Although many of the patients presenting with this illness are desperately ill and will be operated upon hurriedly, it should be borne in mind that,

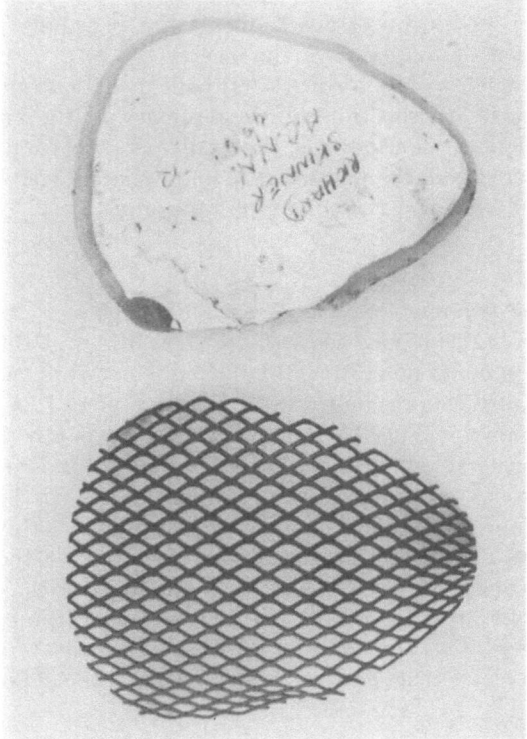

Fig. 17. Bone flap from the same case as Figs. 16 and 3, and the titanium mesh cranioplasty modelled upon it

particularly in frontal sinus cases in the youthful, a perfect cosmetic result should be sought from the beginning. A few minutes preparation at the start may make an excellent cosmetic result possible. Otherwise if the bone is removed piecemeal and no cast is taken of the skull a later cranioplasty is unlikely to be perfect.

Many neurosurgeons will have an established and satisfactory routine for cranioplasty. The following description is of methods which have been developed for the fabrication of titanium mesh or plate based upon the bone removed at the time of craniotomy. If it is intended to discard the bone multiple burr holes may be used. After starting these with a perforator but before enlarging them, an external cast is often extremely useful. It may be made with acrylic resin or dental stent (hard wax with a softening point around 60 °C usually used for dental impressions). Such a cast may be taken in any cases where it is suspected that the bone will be discarded either because of osteomyelitis or brain swelling. The cast should be taken from the skull surface over all the flap to be discarded and beyond the edge of the proposed removal including any other part which may need to be removed such as the eyebrow ridge (Fig. 18). With the aid of this external cast the technician who makes the prosthesis can fill up the burr holes,

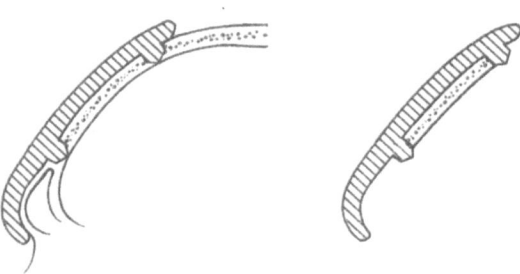

Fig. 18. If the bone is osteomyelitic in the region of the sinuses an external cast may be taken to assist in the fabrication of a perfect cranioplasty. If the external cast is made after the perforator has been used then perfect "keying" of the external cast and the bone will result. This will then assist in locating the bone for accurate building up of it's edge with wax

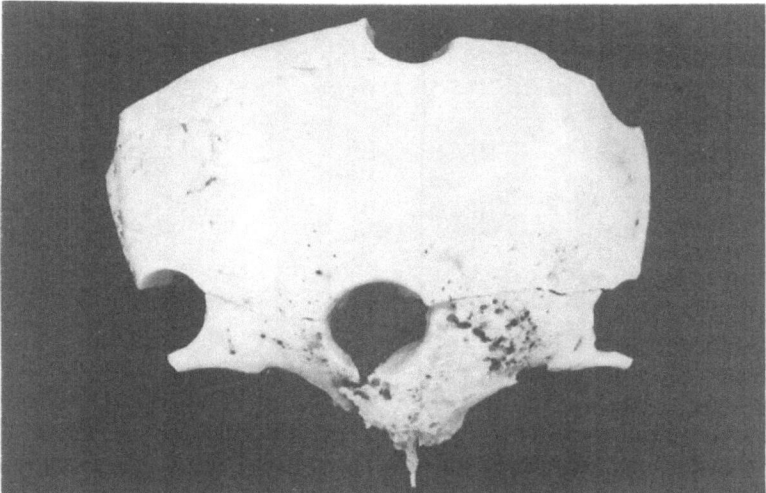

Fig. 19. In cases with very extensive osteomyelitis destroying the inner margins of the eyebrow ridges or the bridge of the nose removal of bone may be thorough. If the pieces are carefully cut so as to leave the maximum amount of bone along the eyebrow ridge then a perfect cranioplasty may be fabricated. This bone was removed in three fragments. They have been glued together prior to filling up the burr holes with wax and extending the edges of the bone flap as shown in Fig. 17

make a wax extension for a few mm beyond the edge of the flap all round with a special extension over the eyebrow if requested, and, using this extended bone flap (Fig. 17) a perfectly fitting mesh or plate can be fabricated. This may be inserted some months later usually with a gratifying result. Titanum is cheap, non-reactive, light and strong and permits radiographic pictures including TCAT scans after insertion. Illustrations of the results using this type of technique are given by Williams (1981).

Post-Operative Management

Even if there have been no attacks before craniotomy there are likely to be fits afterwards and prophyllactic anticonvulsants must be given. Appropriate antibiotics must be continued in adequate dosage. Craniotomy for an infected skull may cause much loss of blood and the patient should be transfused up to normal haemoglobin levels in the anticipation of a possibly necessary second craniotomy.

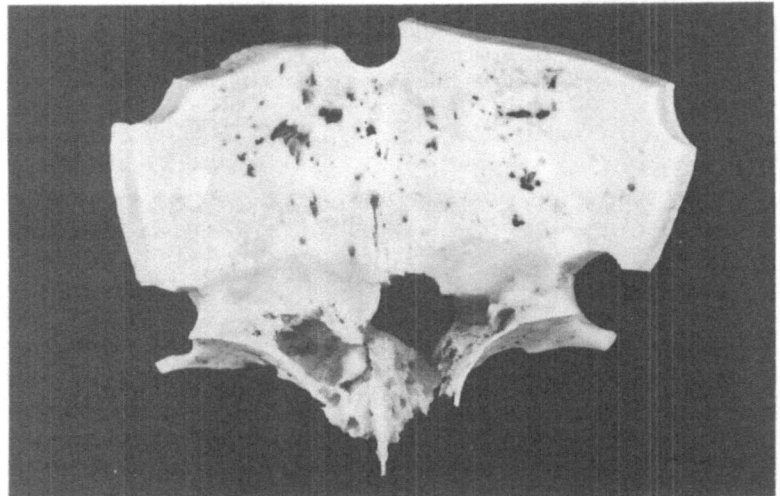

Fig. 20. Back view of the bone removed and shown in Fig. 19

Repeated TCAT scans are of the greatest value in observing the resolution of oedema and the expansion of collections that may have been missed at the first operation. The surgeon should be keen to re-intervene rather than hesitant.

If venous sinus thrombosis is present it is tempting to give anticoagulant treatment by a regime of heparinization or prothrombin inhibition by drugs such as warfarin. The efficacy of such treatment cannot be attested by our clinical results but peripheral oedema and brain swelling may appear to go down more quickly than had been anticipated if anticoagulants are used.

Complications

When spread of pus is extensive it is difficult to decide where it appeared first. So far as possible we have excluded cases of SDE occurring after cerebral abscess as a surgical complication. Of the 90 cases 12 had diagnosable meningitis (11 lived, 1 died) 17 had thrombophlebitis (7 lived, 10 died), 6 had osteomyelitis (4 lived. 2 died), 6 had parenchymatous abscess (2 lived; 3 cerebral and 1 cerebellar abscesses died) and 3 cases had ventriculitis at post-mortem. One survivor had a severe hydrocephalus with associated mental deficit and disinhibition. Clearly the diagnosis of thrombophlebitis was most easily made at necropsy and was probably present much more frequently than these figures suggest. The same may be true of ventriculitis and parenchymatous abscess. Some of our cases had other problems such as renal failure, osteomyelitis elsewhere or congenital heart disease. Because of the poor condition of our hospital records it seems likely that all the complications are underestimated in these figures.

Table 6. *Surgical Treatment, Source of Infection and Mortality*

	Burr Holes						Craniotomy					
	Lived			Died			Lived			Died		
	P	O	M	P	O	M	P	O	M	P	O	M
Primary operation	7	4	1	2	7	3	21	4	1	1	1	0
Secondary operation	7	1	1	2	1	0	15	2	2	3	2	0
Totals by source	14	5	2	4	8	3	36	6	3	4	3	1
	21			15			45			8		

P = Paranasal, O = Otogenic, M = Miscellaneous.

Necropsy Findings

Of the MCNN/BCH cases 14 of the deaths have been examined post-mortem. All of them had residual pus except one of the otogenic group who died with hypertensive glomerulonephritis. Bilateral pus was found in three of the paranasal sinus cases, around the basal cisterns, the suboccipital region and at the convexity in each of the other three. Of the four remaining otogenic cases two had basal pus, one had convexity suppuration and another pus in the cerebello-pontine angle. Residual pus was found in three of the miscellaneous group.

Of the five deaths reported by Anagnostopoulos and Gortvai (1973) four had pus alongside the falx as did one of the cases of Hitchcock and Andreadis (1964).

Mortality

In the present series mortality does not correlate closely with age but the patients in the first and second decade had a mortality of 6 out of 45 (13%) with impaired survival in the other groups. Paranasal infections had a better outcome than the others (P < 0.1). The paranasal mortality was 8 out of 58 with 11 out of 22 in the otogenic group (Table 6). Aerobic streptococci in the isolates was another favourable feature (Table 3) as was a long history and female sex. The significance of the long history is that such cases were less fulminating in onset.

The overwhelming feature about the mortality however, was the superior results obtained by craniotomy (Table 6). In this table cases in which exploratory burr holes were followed by immediate craniotomy are designated as primary craniotomy. Third and fourth operations are treated as second operations. If craniotomy was decided upon initially the survival rate was 26 cases out of 28 (93%) and for secondary craniotomy it was 19 cases out of 24 (80%). The survival of those cases treated by burr holes was 21 out of 36 (58%). This striking finding was anticipated by many authors. The paper of Kubik and Adams (1943) stated "Surgical treatment should consist of drainage through a lateral frontal craniotomy and not through the frontal sinus or mastoidectomy wound. Performed in this way, the operation is simple and quick and, if the results are negative, little or no harm is done". Similar advice came from Glass (1947), Stern and Boldrey (1952), Torres, Yarzagaray and West (1975) and Borzone, Capuzzo and Rivano (1980). Several authors however have failed to appreciate the importance of craniotomy and some have advised against it. Clearly the factors which lead Gardner to advise against running the risks of spreading infection in 1933 are, in an antibiotic age, no longer operative. A waiting policy in the hope of improved localisation has little to commend it. In more modern series the chief factors leading to failure to recognise the importance of craniotomy seem to have been the smallness of the series of patients accumulated and the straightforward acceptance of someone else's statement that burr holes and local antibiotics *is* the treatment. Schiller, Cairns and Russell (1948) appear to have been responsible for this view.

Since the publication of Bannister *et al.* (1981) it has been clear that craniotomy and craniectomy give an improved chance of survival. Table 6 presents an update of Bannister's figures. Infants treated by fontanelle aspiration have been excluded, attempts at clearance through a mastoid cavity have been included in the burr hole group. Not all reports are suitable for analysis in such a table, reports of multiple trephinations (Farmer and Wise 1973, Reynaudin and Frazee 1980, Despert *et al.* 1981) are difficult to categorise. Other reports, particularly describing intracranial sepsis in general, are sometimes insufficiently specific (McLaurin 1969, Garfield 1969, Galbraith and Barr 1974, Kaufman 1975). Recent reports from Tovi *et al.* (1980) and Hatanaka *et al.* (1981) have not been included.

Considering mortality alone, and reviewing the data given in Table 7 it is clear that craniotomy is a significantly better treatment than burr holes (P < 0.01). If cases treated at MCNN since Bannister's analysis are added by substituting data from Table 6 for Bannister and Hockley the figures look very convincing. Treatments designed to remove all pus under direct vision, that is counting craniectomy and craniotomy both primary and secondary together, the cases total 164 with a mortality of 21 (15%) as opposed to burr hole treatment cases totalling 238 with a mortality of 74 (31%). This analysis includes cases of secondary craniotomy, that is to say, a proportion of cases that were initially wrongly treated by burr holes. In this group of 37 cases the mortality was 10 (27%) and if they are excluded, the primary/craniectomy group of 127 cases had a mortality of only 13 (10%). Comparing this again with the 31%

Table 7. *Combined Literature of the Antibiotic Era*

Author	No of Cases	Primary Craniotomy		Secondary Craniotomy		Craniectomy + Local Antibiotics		Burr Holes + Local Antibiotics		Burr Holes Alone	
		L	D	L	D	L	D	L	D	L	D
Gross (1946)	1					1					
Anderson (1947)	1					1					
Glass (1947)	1	1									
Schiller (1948)	10			1				6	3		
Gurdjian (1948)	4							3		1	
Keith (1949)	7					3		2		2	
Le Beau (1949)	7	6	1								
List (1950)	1			1							
Botterell (1952)	9					9					
Stern (1952)	7					6	1				
Wood (1952)	11							6	4	1	
Jacobson (1954)	1			1							
List (1955)	2					2					
Biehl (1955)	1						1				
Stephens (1956)	1									1	
Niebeling (1959)	2								1	1	
Genest (1963)	1	1									
Hitchcock (1964)	29							19	7		3
Mincy (1966)	1	1									
Woodhall (1967)	10	1						5	4		
Hollin (1967)	3			1		1					1
Murphy (1968)	1	1									
Whittam (1969)	3	1		1							1
Beeden (1969)	2									2	
Torres (1970)	13	9			1					1	2
Weinman (1972)	47							35	12		
Coonrod (1972)	7							2		3	2
Anagnostopoulos (1973)	32							27	5		
Le Beau (1973)	37	20	6	1	4			2	4		
Osgood (1975)	1	1									
Verdura (1975)	2	2									
Van Alphen (1976)	18									12	6
Pelc (1976)	2	2									
Joubert (1977)	7	1						4	2		
Van Dellen (1977)	5	2								3	
Swaiman (1977)	1	1									
Stephanov (1979)	7			2				3	2		
Borzone (1980)	14	10	2					2			
Luken (1980)	4	4									
Bannister (1981)	66	21	2	13	3					13	14
Hockley (1982)	4			4							
Totals		85	11	25	8	23	2	116	44	40	29

L = Lived, D = Died.

mortality for burr hole treatment it seems likely that the chances of survival are increased by a factor of close to 3 if the initial treatment is energetic craniotomy rather than burr holes.

Obviously, delay in diagnosis is a factor of paramount importance in management. Galbraith and Barr (1974) found that 7 out of their 21 cases died before being seen by a neurosurgeon. It is generally agreed that this is a universally fatal condition unless treated by surgery although obviously such a statement cannot be tested. It is necessary for neurosurgeons to provide continuing education to neurologists, physicians and particularly paediatricians whose chance to see such cases is necessarily less than the opportunities which occur in busy neurosurgery units.

Morbidity

With such a dire disease carrying so high a mortality and from the dismal appearance at the height of the illness with fits, hemiparesis and unconsciousness it might be anticipated that a severe morbidity would commonly result. Weinman and Samarasinghe (1972) observed that "the vast majority" of their 75% survival made a complete recovery with no neurological deficit. Anagnostopoulos and Gortvai (1973) commented that 16 of their 27 survivors had post-operative fits 1-2 years after operation. Hitchcock and Andreadis (1964) found that out of 19 survivors only 5 (26%) had fits after three years in a review of the 12 patients who had come to follow-up for longer than that period. One patient had her first fit five years after the illness. Borzone *et al.* (1980) followed 8 of their 12 survivors for 3 years or more, 3 of these had epilepsy and one had a persisting hemiplegia.

Of the MCNN/BCH cases totalling 90 there were 66 survivors (73%) and the patients upon whom there is an adequate follow-up of twelve months or more total 50.

Neurological Deficits

Hemianopia was present in 17 of the cases at the zenith of the illness and ophthalmoplegia in 21. No survivor retained hemianopia but one still had an ophthalmoplegia 23 years later. (Table 8).

Hemiparesis was present in the acute stage in 62 of the acute patients and was a persisting problem in 9 out of 50 traced survivors, it was not so severe as to interfere with mobility in any late case.

Dysphasia was present in 16 of the presenting cases but persisted in only two of the 50. Only two survivors had an egregious intellectual deficit.

Epilepsy

Epileptic seizures were present in 56 of the acute illnesses. Epilepsy in the acute stage did not correlate with survival nor does it correlate significantly with late epilepsy (Table 9). This contrasts with the findings of Anagnostopoulos and

Table 8. *Origin of Sepsis and Neurological Deficit in Survivors*

		Early (N = 54)				Late (N = 42)			
	Nos	Epi-lepsy	Dys-phasia	Hemi-paresis	Hemi-anopia	Epi-lepsy	Dys-phasia	Hemi-paresis	Hemi-anopia
Paranasal	39	30	10	32	8	10	0	5	0
Otogenic	10	1	0	4	1	1	1	1	0
Other	5	4	0	1	0	0	0	0	0

Table 9. *Early Epilepsy and the Incidence of Late Fits*

Epilepsy status in the acute illness	(N = 60)	Total seen at follow up (N = 50)	No fits	Type of late fit			
				Focal	Generalised	Both	Total
No fits	21	18	11	0	7	0	7
Focal fits	24	20	13	3	2	2	7
Generalised fits	7	6	5	0	1	0	1
Both kinds of fit	8	6	5	1	0	0	1

Gortvai (1973) that epilepsy was three times commoner in the late stages of cases who had fits before operation. As expected, epilepsy was commoner in the younger age groups both early and late but this fell outside significance level (P > 0.05). Paranasal sinusitis was more likely to give early fits than other causes (P < 0.01) but the apparent difference in the incidence of late seizures resulting therefrom was not significant (Table 8). No relationship was found between the worst level of consciousness and either early or late seizures. The occurrence of fits related to treatment has been given in Table 4. There was no observable lessening of epilepsy if craniotomy was used, 10 of the 31 craniotomy cases followed up had late epilepsy as opposed to 5 of the 14 cases treated by burr holes. Of the 60 who survived with adequate records, 50 have adequate follow up and 16 of these late epilepsy (Cowie and Williams 1982). This is most commonly not socially disabling. In one case the epilepsy was sufficiently severe to justify late craniotomy and frontal lobe removal but the result was only an improvement in the number of daily fits.

Of the 18 patients who had no epilepsy in the acute stage and had adequate follow up, seven patients developed late epilepsy (Table 9). The fits came on within 16 months in 5 of these 7 and in the other two the first fits were at 4 and 5 years respectively.

Discussion

Because SDE has always been, and remains, a rare disease individual surgeons are unlikely to see more than a handful of cases in a lifetime. Referrals are likely to be dealt with by inexperienced residents or other junior staff and it seems to be important to make the condition known to them before they see their first case rather than afterwards. Because of the rarity of the condition neurosurgeons are the only doctors likely to see a significant number of cases and this places them in an important position for maintaining awareness of the disease and for acting promptly when it is suspected. When confronted by a patient who is extremely ill it may be tempting to forgo a craniotomy. The suggestion might be made that the marked improvement in results from craniotomy as opposed to burr holes reported by Bannister et al. (1981) and re-reported here, was due to patient selection. Table 4 shows that in the two worst groupings craniotomy was used more often than burr holes but proportionately not so frequently as in the two best groupings. This preference was not statistically significant.

Because of the rarity of the condition realisation of the advantages of craniotomy has come only slowly to this centre, the report of Bhandari and Sarkari from MCNN did not note the advantages of craniotomy as recently as 1970. At the present it seems almost certain that the improvement in mortality reflected by Fig. 2 has been due to the greater readiness to practice early craniotomy in the MCNN.

An alternative interpretation might be that the greater variety of antibiotics presently available gives some advantage. Antibiotic resistance does not seem to be a problem however, no chloramphenicol resistant strain has been isolated in this series and some of the most impressive results reported, such as the cases of Botterell and Drake (1952) and Stern and Boldrey (1952) relied mostly on penicillin.

The availability of TCAT scanning to monitor complications such as enlargement of residual collections of pus, hydrocephalus and development of parenchymatous abscess (Joubert and Stephanov 1977) has certainly made the management of these cases easier; although it may not have made initial diagnosis more rapidly or reliably than previous methods.

The management of survivors in respect of epilepsy may be debated. Hitchcock and Andreadis (1964) say that their experience of one third of their surviving cases having epilepsy lead them to advise that all cases should have anticonvulsants for "an indefinite period". At the end of the first 3 years however, only 3 of their cases were following this advice. Alternative advice might be based on the view that, independent of the fit status in the acute stage, about two thirds of the patients will have no epilepsy after recovery from the acute stage of the illness. The sooner it is decided whether or not the patient is going to be an established epileptic the better it is for the patient. If they have had a fit then there is no doubt that they have the incentive to continue with anticonvulsants and the reassurance that such treatment is justifiable. Many of the patients are children of school age and it is better for them to have a fit at school rather than have the first seizure after having started work or having taken up driving. Because of these considerations the author has changed his practice from an enthusiastic advocate of a routine anticonvulsants and has not had occasion to regret the policy of weaning off anticonvulsants six or eight weeks after return home.

Conclusions

Subdural empyema is a fierce illness affecting most commonly the young. It has a rapidly progressive course with more obvious signs of infection than most septic illnesses, the most common findings including sinusitis, drowsiness, meningism, pyrexia, hemiplegia and epilepsy. The natural course is of rapid downhill progression and death but in almost no other condition is immediate and radical craniotomy more likely to produce an excellent result. Attempts at treatments at treatment by burr holes alone and the addition of antibiotics to the intracranial volume by instillation are no longer acceptable. Although they are uncommon cases, widespread knowledge leading to early recognition of the condition and understanding of the correct lines of treatment may produce excellent rewards. An awareness that bone may need to be removed and that the patients are likely to survive should lead to planning for likely cranioplasty from the start of the illness. Longstanding neurological sequelae are uncommon and late epilepsy occurs in only about one third of survivors. Prophyllactic anticonvulsants are therefore not necessary after the resolution of the acute illness.

Acknowledgements

My colleagues G. Bannister, R. Cowie, C. Hilton, and S. Smith have been invaluable in analysing the MCNN records and I am grateful to Mr. A. D. Hockley for data from the BCH. Mr. J. Marsden has made the titanium mesh prostheses illustrated.

References

Anagnostopoulos, D. I., Gortvai, P., 1973: Intracranial subdural abscess. Brit. J. Surg. *60*, 50—52.

Anderson, F. M., 1947: Subdural empyema secondary to frontal sinusitis. Review of clinical features and report of three cases. Ann. Otol. Rhinol. Laryngol. *56*, 5—17.

Van Alphen, H. A. M., Dreissen, J. J. R. 1976: Brain abscess and subdural empyema. Factors influencing mortality and results of various surgical techniques. J. Neurol. Neurosurg. Psychiat. *39*, 481—490.

Bannister, G., Williams, B., Smith, S., 1981: Treatment of subdural empyema. J. Neurosurg. *55*, 82—88.

Beeden, A. G., Marsden, C. D., Meadows, J. C., Michael, W. F., 1969: Intracranial complications of middle ear disease and mastoid surgery. J. Neurol. Sci. *9*, 261—272.

Bell, W. E., McCormick, W. F., 1975: Neurologic infections in children, pp. 47—48. Philadelphia: Saunders.

Bhandari, Y. S., Sarkari, N. B. S., 1970: Subdural empyema. A review of 37 cases. J. Neurosurg. *32*, 35—39.

Biehl, J. P., 1955: Subdural empyema secondary to acute frontal sinusitis. A neglected but curable emergency complication. J. A. M. A. *158*, 721—724.

Borzone, M., Capuzzo, T., Rivano, C., Tortori-Donati, P., 1980: Subdural empyema: fourteen cases surgically treated. Surg. Neurol. *13*, 449—452.

Botterell, E. H., Drake, C. G., 1952: Localised encephalitis, brain abscess and subdural empyema. J. Neurosurg. *9*, 348—366.

Coonrod, J. D., Dans, P. E., 1972: Subdural empyema. Amer. J. Med. *53*, 85—91.

Courville, C. B., 1944: Subdural empyema secondary to purulent frontal sinusitis. A clinicopathological study of forty-two cases verified at autopsy. Arch. Otolaryngol. *39*, 211—230.

Cowie, R., Williams, B., 1982: Morbidity after subdural empyema. In preparation.

Delgado-Escueta, A. V., Wasterlain, C., Treiman, D. M., Porter, R. J., 1982: Management of status epilepticus. N. Eng. J. Med. *306*, 1337—1340.

Van Dellen, J. R., Boles, D. M., Van Den Heever, C. M., 1977: Interhemispheric subdural empyema. S. Afr. Med. J. *52*, 266—269.

Despert, F., Santini, J. J., Ployet, M. J., Chantepie, A., Fauchier, Cl., Combe, P., 1981: L'empyème sous-dural: Une complication rare des infections O. R. L. chez l'enfant. Ann. Paediat. *28*, 591—595.

Dumville, A. W., 1858: Remarks in trephining the skull. Illustrated by a case. Brit. Med. J. *2*, 743.

Farmer, T. W., Wise, G. R., 1973: Subdural empyema in infants, children and adults. Neurology *23*, 254—261.

Galbraith, J. G., Barr, V. W., 1974: Epidural abscess and subdural empyema, In: Infectious Diseases of the Central Nervous System. Advances in Neurology, Vol. 6 (Thompson, R. A., Green, J. R., eds.), pp. 257—267. New York: Raven Press.

Gardner, W. J., 1933: Subdural abscess in relation to sterile purulent leptomeningitis. Ohio State Med. J. *29*, 235—238.

Garfield, J., 1969: Management of supratentorial intracranial abscess: a review of 200 cases. Brit. Med. J. *2*, 7—11.

Genest, A. S., Bingham, W. G., Hamilton, R. D., 1963: Bilateral subdural empyema. Report of case with arteriograms. J. Neurosurg. *20*, 524—526.

Glass, R. L., 1947: Osteoplastic flap method in treatment of subdural abscess. J. Neurosurg. *4*, 391—393.

Griffith, H. B., 1968: Factors in the mortality of cerebellar abscess. J. Neurol. Neurosurg. Psychiat. *31*, 89.

Gross, S. W., 1873: An examination of the causes, diagnosis and operative treatment of compression of the brain, as met with in Army practice. Amer. J. Med. Sci. *66*, 40—74.

— 1946: Osteomyelitis of the frontal bone and subdural empyema with recovery. Amer. J. Surg. *71*, 828—831.

Gurdjian, E. S., Thomas, L. M., 1969: Surgical treatment of cranial and intracranial suppuration. Springfield: Thomas.

— Webster, J. E., 1948: Modern surgical treatment of acute subdural abscess. Arch. Surg. *57*, 411—426.

Hankinson, J., Amador, L. V., 1956: Infected subdural effusions. Brit. Med. J. *11*, 122—126.

Hatanaka, M., Ishii, M., Oda, N., Iwabuchi, T., 1981: Multiple subdural abscess including one in the interhemisphere. No Shinkei Geka *9*, 1053—1058.

Hilton, C. M., 1981: Twelve year review of intracranial abscesses. Personal communication.

Hitchcock, E., Andreadis, A., 1964: Subdural empyema: a review of 29 cases. J. Neurol. Neurosurg. Psychiat. *27*, 422—434.

Hockley, A. D., 1982: Personal communication.

Hollin, S. A., Hayashi, H., Gross, S. W., 1967: Intracranial abscesses of odontogenic origin. Oral Surg. *23*, 277—293.

Jacobson, S. A., Kane, C. A., 1954: Purulent subdural collection. Neurology *4*, 558—562.

Jefferson, G., 1947: The surgery of intracranial abscess. In: Modern Operative Surgery (Turner, G. G., ed.), pp. 1266—1273. London: Cassell.

Joubert, M. J., Stephanov, S., 1977: Computerized tomography and surgical treatment in intracranial suppuration. Report of 30 consecutive unselected cases of brain abscess and subdural empyema. J. Neurosurg. *47*, 73—78.

Kalbag, R. M., Woolf, A. L., 1967: Cerebral venous thrombosis. London-New York-Toronto: Oxford U. P.

Kaufman, D. M., Miller, M. H., Steigbigel, N. H., 1975: Subdural empyema; analysis of 17 recent cases and review of the literature. Medicine *54*, 485—498.

Keith, W. S., 1949: Subdural empyema. J. Neurosurg. *6*, 127—139.

Kiser, J. L., Kendig, J. H., 1963: Intracranial suppuration. A review of 139 consecutive cases with electron-microscopic observations on three. J. Neurosurg. *20*, 494—511.

Klastersky, J., Kahan-Coppens, L., Brihaye, J., 1979: Infections in neurosurgery. In: Advances and Technical Standards in Neurosurgery, Vol. 6 (Krayenbühl, H., *et al.* eds.), pp. 39—54. Wien-New York: Springer.

Kubik, C. S., Adams, R. D., 1943: Subdural empyema. Brain *68*, 18—42.

La Peyronie, F. G. De, 1744: Hist. dé L'Acad. Roy. des Sciences. Sabatier, Médecine Opératoire, p. 212.

Le Beau, J., 1949: Traitement chirurgical de l'empyème sous-dural et sous-arachnoidien. Rev. Neurol. *81*, 828—851.

— Creissard, P., Harispe, L., Redondo, A., 1973: Surgical treatment of brain abscess and subdural empyema. J. Neurosurg. *38*, 198—203.

List, C. F., 1950: Interhemispheral subdural suppuration. J. Neurosurg. *7*, 313—324.

— 1955: Diagnosis and treatment of acute subdural empyema. Neurology *5*, 663—670.

Luken, M. G. III., Whelan, M. A., 1980: Recent diagnostic experience with subdural empyema. J. Neurosurg. *52*, 764—771.

Macewen, W., 1893: Pyogenic diseases of the brain and spinal cord. Glasgow: McLehose.

McLaurin, R. L., 1969: Subdural infection. In: Surgical treatment of cranial and intracranial suppuration (Gurdjian, E. S., Thomas, L. M., eds.), pp. 73—88. Springfield: Thomas.

Milhorat, T. H., 1978: Peadiatric Neurosurgery. Philadelphia: Davis.

Mincy, J. E., Peck, F. C. Jr., 1966: Actinomycotic subdural empyema. Survival following surgical draining and antibiotic treatment. N. Y. State J. Med. *66*, 2155—2157.

Murphy, J. P., Wilkes, J. D., 1968: Subdural abscess diagnosed by brain scanning. South Med. J. *61*, 564—611.

Niebeling, H. G., 1959: Subdural empyema. Neurochirurgia *2*, 47—54.

Northfield, D. W. C., 1973: The surgery of the central nervous system. Oxford: Blackwell.

Osgood, C. P., Dujovny, M., Holm, E., Postic, B., 1975: Delayed post-traumatic subdural empyema. J. Trauma *15*, 916—921.

Pelc, S., 1976: Subdural empyema. Acta Univ. Carol. (Med. Monogr.) *75*, 174—175.

Pool, J. L., Potanos, J. N., Krueger, E. G., 1962: Osteomas and mucocoeles of the frontal paranasal sinuses. J. Neurosurg. *19*, 130—135.

Post, E. M., Modesti, L. M., 1981: "Subacute" post operative subdural empyema. J. Neurosurg. *55*, 761—765.

Purdom, D. R., Salmon, M. V., Williams, B., 1976: False positive immuno-fluorescence test for herpes simplex in tuberculous meningitis. Lancet *1*, 1235—1236.

Reynaudin, J. W., Frazee, J., 1980: Subdural empyema — importance of early diagnosis. Neurosurgery *7*, 477—479.

Schiller, F., Cairns, H., Russell, D. S., 1948: Treatment of purulent pachymeningitis and subdural suppuration with special reference to penicillin. J. Neurol. Neurosurg. Psychiat. *11*, 143—182.

Stephanov, S., Joubert, M. J., Welchman, J. M., 1979: Combined convexity and parafalx subdural empyema. Surg. Neurol. *11*, 147—151.

Stephens, J., Welch, K., 1956: Subdural abscess with retinal thrombophlebitis. Neurology *6*, 889—890.

Stern, W. E., Boldrey, E., 1952: Subdural purulent collections. Surg. Gynec. Obstet. *95*, 623—630.

Swaiman, K. F., Gold, L. H. A., 1977: An unusual computed tomographic appearance of a subdural empyema. J. Pediatr. *91*, 945—947.

Torres, H., Yarzagaray, L., West, C., 1970: Subdural empyema, angiographic and clinic considerations. Neurochirurgia *13*, 201—210.

Tovi, F., Sidi, Z., Cohen, A., Tribron, P., 1980: Subdural empyema complicating acute paranasal sinusitis. Harefuah. *99*, 371—373.

Verdura, J., White, R. J., Resnikoff, S., *et al.* 1975: Interhemispheric subdural empyema; angiographic diagnosis and surgical treatment. Surg. Neurol. *3*, 89—92.

Watson, P. H., 1870: Case of intracranial abscess following injury successfully treated by trephining. Edinb. Med. J. *16*, 43.

Weinman, D., Samarasinghe, H. H. R., 1972: Subdural empyema. Aust. NZ. J. Surg. *41*, 324—330.

Whittam, D. E., Pickard, B. H., Wilson, T. D. H., 1968: Brain abscess and otitis media. Acta Otorhinolaryngol. Belg. *23*, 375—383.

Williams, B., 1981: Subdural empyema. Hospital Update *8*, 111—126.

— 1982: The neurosurgery of oto-rhinological sepsis. Clin. Otolaryngol., in press.

Wood, P. H., 1952: Diffuse subdural suppuration. J. Laryngol. Otol. *66*, 496—515.

Woodhall, B., 1967: Osteomyelitis and epi-, extra-, and subdural abscesses. Clin. Neurosurg. *14*, 239—255.

Wright, R. L., 1969: Septic complications of intracranial surgery. In: Surgical treatment of cranial and intracranial suppuration (Gurdjian, E. S., Thomas, L. M., eds.), pp. 93—112. Springfield: Thomas.

Yoshikawa, T. T., Chow, A. W., Guze, L. B., 1975: Role of anaerobic bacteria in subdural empyema. Report of four cases and review of 327 cases from the English literature. Amer. J. Med. *58*, 99—104.

Author Index

Subject Index

Advances and Technical Standards in Neurosurgery

Editors: H. Krayenbühl (Managing Editor),
J. Brihaye, F. Loew, V. Logue, S. Mingrino, B. Pertuiset,
L. Symon, H. Troupp, M. G. Yaşargil

Volume 8

1981. 135 partly coloured figures.
XII, 328 pages.
ISBN 3-211-81665-8

Volume 7

1980. 147 figures. XI, 247 pages.
ISBN 3-211-81592-9

Volume 6

1979. 79 figures. XI, 191 pages.
ISBN 3-211-81518-X

Volume 5

1978. 78 figures. XII, 224 pages.
ISBN 3-211-81441-8

Volume 4

1977. 66 partly coloured figures.
XI, 154 pages.
ISBN 3-211-81423-X

Volume 3

1976. 77 figures. XI, 154 pages.
ISBN 3-211-81381-0

Volume 2

1975. 150 partly coloured figures.
XI, 217 pages.
ISBN 3-211-81293-8

Volume 1

1974. 96 figures. XI, 210 pages.
ISBN 3-211-81218-0

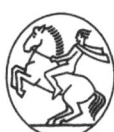

Springer-Verlag Wien New York